Resilience and Military Families

This textbook aims to educate students across all mental health disciplines on the importance of using strengths-based resilience as a tool when working with military families. Organized into three main sections using the military deployment cycle, including the stages of pre-deployment, deployment, and post-deployment, this textbook examines some of the key resiliency skills that operate in military families so that students can understand how many families not only survive, but learn how to thrive, despite great challenges.

Chapters address the military family at home, resilient family systems, the importance of effective communication and social support, the impact of trauma and moral injury, and the transition from military to civilian life following service. Filled with case vignettes, self-assessment tools, and evidence-informed interventions, readers learn multiple ways to measure, assess, and strengthen family resiliency throughout the book. In addition to these skills, specific examples are highlighted that draw lessons from the military community on stress management and posttraumatic growth in the context of family life. The book finishes with an appendix that includes suggestions for therapists on the use of cultural humility to improve treatment.

Following two decades of war and a global pandemic, this essential textbook is a crucial read for all mental health professionals training to work with military-connected populations and their families. Professionals from disciplines including clinical social work, marriage and family therapy, psychology, healthcare, and theology as well as instructors of courses on military social work, military psychology, and mental health will all find this text an invaluable resource.

Julie Canfield, PhD, LICSW, is a clinical instructor at Boston College School for Social Work and maintains a private practice in Boston, Massachusetts, dedicated to providing effective mental health treatment to active-duty service members, military veterans, military-connected children, and families impacted by military service. Dr. Canfield is the military spouse of a combat veteran and holds a doctorate in social work from Smith College School of Social Work. Her research career has focused on improving clinical treatment and practices for childhood trauma, secondary traumatization in family systems, and improving professional resilience among child and family trauma therapists. Dr. Canfield holds a master's degree in social work from Hunter College of the City University of New York and a bachelor's degree from New York University.

Resilience and Military Families

Case Vignettes, Self-Assessment Tools, and Evidence-Based Interventions

Julie Canfield

Routledge
Taylor & Francis Group
NEW YORK AND LONDON

Designed cover image: © Getty Images

First published 2025
by Routledge
605 Third Avenue, New York, NY 10158

and by Routledge
4 Park Square, Milton Park, Abingdon, Oxon OX14 4RN

Routledge is an imprint of the Taylor & Francis Group, an informa business

ISBN: 978-1-032-57177-5 (hbk)
ISBN: 978-1-032-57176-8 (pbk)
ISBN: 978-1-003-43822-9 (ebk)

DOI: 10.4324/9781003438229

Typeset in Sabon
by Taylor & Francis Books

This book is dedicated to the hundreds of thousands of children who did not choose the military life, but live it every day with a silent dignity and integrity that few ever imagine. Thank you for showing up when it is needed the most. Thank you for not complaining for all of your sacrifices. Thank you for holding onto hope for your family. Thank you for shining light into darkness ... and thank you for your service!

Contents

List of Illustrations viii

Introduction 1

PART 1
Pre-Deployment Resiliency: "The Calm Before the Storm" 5

1 Military Family Culture 7

2 Resiliency in the Military Family 31

3 Assessing Family Capacity to Manage Stress 47

PART 2
Deployment Resiliency: "Managing the Storm" 57

4 Military Families Adapting to Stress 59

5 Attachment Disruptions and Coping Strategies 73

6 Trauma, Attachment, and Treatment Interventions 92

PART 3
Post-Deployment Resiliency: "Assessing the Effects of the Storm" 107

7 Posttraumatic Stress in Military Family Life 109

8 Injuries of War and the Military Family 125

9 Military Families Transition to Civilian Life 136

Appendix 152
Bibliography 160
Index 170

Illustrations

Figures

1.1 Social characteristics of the fortress, warrior society: characteristics, and psychological characteristics of the fortress 22
1.2 Cultural competency vs. cultural humility 25
2.1 Military spouses: protective (+) and risk (-) factors 35
2.2 The 5 Cs of Positive Youth Development (PYD) Model (Lerner et al., 2018) 44
4.1 The double ABCX model of family adaptation to stress (McCubbin and Patterson, 1983) 63
6.1 Overlap of PTSD and PPCS symptoms 95
6.2 Co-occurring mental health concerns 95
6.3 Trauma and attachment 101
6.4 Trauma/attachment and emotions 102
6.5 Trauma/attachment and resilience 102
6.6 Attachment styles in relationships (Bowlby & Ainsworth, 2013) 102
7.1 Interactional cycle of cascading effects in the family system with potential outcomes during reintegration phase following high-stress military deployment in at-risk families. (Potential effects illustrated through the lens of the double ABCX model of family adaptation to stress of McCubbin & Patterson, 1983). 121
7.2 Role confusion and boundary ambiguity in secondary traumatic stress 122
7.3 Secondary traumatic stress 124

Boxes

Case Example 29
Families Responding to Notification Orders (Case Study) 46
Parenting Challenges (Case Example) 71
Family Adjustment and Adaptation to Stress Model (Case Example) 89
Solution-Focused Brief Therapy (Case Example) 104
Environmental and Internal Triggers of Traumatic Stress 124
Military Medical Retirements (Case Example) 134
Veterans and Civilian Employment Challenges (Case Example) 150

Introduction

"Thank you for your service." The response is usually a smile, a shrug, a nod ... very rarely a spoken response because what is there to say to this comment other than "you're welcome" which is often unexpected and misinterpreted as a result. These communications are often fleeting and superficial but we would never want to live without them. We agree as a society to have a military and count on there being enough young adults who voluntarily sign up for military service so that we never resort to conscription again. We agree to support and sustain our military but do so hoping that there is no war for them to fight. Sadly however, each generation has its war (or wars), and the long ones begin before many of the new military recruits are born. An entire generation recently grew up with at least one war going on despite the fact that a large portion of U.S. citizens knew few military service members and many could not point to the geographic location for the wars on an unidentified map of the world.

> "My father's never been to any of my basketball games; by the time I got out of elementary school, my mother had deployed three times and we had lived in six locations across two continents. When they were home they didn't really feel like playing or have the time to hang out and watch my games. When they finally retired from the military, I was 20 years old and had moved out ... grown up and moved out."

Silence.

"Please thank your parents for their service."

A smile, a shrug, a nod.

This is not a book about how strong military families are because they are not any stronger than non-military (civilian) families. They are not any stronger, but many learned how to cope with adversity, adapt to stressful situations, and to endure despite them. They survive because survival is a skill you learn when you need to learn it. Military families often have family members who served across multiple generations and resilience was as much a part of intergenerational family life as it was for childhood development. Military families often embrace discipline and a determination to survive by becoming comfortable with self-sacrifice along the way. One military spouse described herself as "scrappy" and explained that although she did not always have the resources to manage certain challenging situations over the course of their family's years of active duty, she was able to overcome these by taking risks and "putting herself out there." She did this through willpower and a drive to do what needed to be done. She explained that she did not have a choice but to reach her family's goals to succeed because "failure was not an option."

The military family in the post-9/11 volunteer force experienced repeated separations of at least one family member to overseas combat deployments and training missions at

DOI: 10.4324/9781003438229-1

home in what has been referred to in military jargon as a period of "high operational tempo." Tempos are considered too high or too low if they place forces at risk of losing their capacity to sustain operations and meet crises. The meaning of this phrase is similar to finding the level of intensity of stress that causes an individual, family, or organization to grow from meeting demands that are not overly taxing the system's capacity to manage and meet those demands. This is sometimes referred to as the place where resiliency grows. The post-9/11 wars had such a high operational tempo that a level was reached for many families that was unsustainable in terms of maintaining individual and family resiliency and truly effective recovery from the related stress.

As the military reorganized following two decades of war, it transitioned waves of service members to veteran status and replaced them with a new generation of younger warriors fit for duty and ready to take on the challenges of military life. This new generation of warriors are recruited in high schools and communities across the country, leaving home, becoming trained in military defense while getting married, having children, and establishing families who will be impacted by the next wave of military service to the country. It would be unwise to lose the lessons we have learned over the course of the past two decades of the longest period in our history of repeated wartime deployments and the impact on families from such demanding and sustained military operations. In an effort to expand the current body of literature beyond the veteran's experience from military service to civilian life, this research began during the height of repetitive deployments (around 2011–2012) when military families were continually responding to what seemed to be the never-ending wars. Military demands were constant and the threat of combat deployments a constant reality that was always possible for service members and their families. Family members had careers, relationships, and childhood developments interrupted as a result and deserve research and policy agendas aimed at supporting military family life regardless of the service member's involvement. While the military organization has the structure in place to regenerate its force by replacement with a new generation to maintain resiliency and strength, the military family does not have that option, and as a result experience the effects of wartime service for generations.

The reintegration process continues to be challenging for many military/veteran families as behavioral health treatments were adapted for veterans from other conditions stemming from trauma that were evidence-based for those conditions and sometimes did more harm than good. Treatments for topics around issues of morality that result from participation in war are still being developed and therapeutic conversations about these topics leave most civilian therapists at a loss in our current cultural climate. Although the risk factors are well known, what to do about them is less so, particularly concerning family conflicts, family dissolution, stress, depression, and suicides among military families. Well-meaning providers often continue to search for ways to take away negative feelings experienced in the military/veteran communities rather than assist families in learning how to manage them and navigate what are often very difficult conversations. The military community in the United States constitutes less than 1% of the total population, from active-duty families to National Guard and Reserve units living most of their time as civilians. The numbers matter because when 99% of an entire population is not impacted by an experience, there is a reduced drive to attempt to understand the complexity of the issues involved, and a gap in collective understanding emerges as a result. The concepts concerning resiliency that are addressed in this book are not limited to military families and the capacity to respond to a stressful situation in a healthy and adaptive manner is a crucial part of any family's life. Military families are called to adapt to change on a regular basis and develop skills for managing stress through affect management that offers insight into resiliency for all families. Adaptations are needed throughout all the phases of military family life with multiple geographic relocations, separations, losses, and additions to family life resulting from these changes (new schools, communities, friends, and workplaces) that are seamlessly all woven into the fabric of daily life. The deployment experience is a stressful situation in family life marked by three distinct periods of adaptation and family functioning: preparing for the event; managing the situation; and then coping with the effects that follow as new identities and family narratives are created that integrate the experience.

This book addresses the resiliency point at which individuals and families have the opportunity to grow from adversity that is stressful, challenging, and demanding of both internal and external resources. It outlines the core ingredients for meeting these demands at this point so that the person or family does not become overwhelmed by an event, situation, or crisis in family life and lose its strength as a result. The resiliency point is that point in time when one reaches a crossroads in managing stress and has choices to make to successfully adapt to it and overcome its challenges or to take a different path. Through education and awareness of these choices, both military and civilian families can learn that there are options for choosing the path toward resiliency because failure is never an option.

Part 1

Pre-Deployment Resiliency

"The Calm Before the Storm"

1 Military Family Culture

Demographic Background

To say that military families in the United States live a unique lifestyle would be an understatement because some aspects of that life defy simple explanations, including entire families that all pack up and move to new geographic locations every few years. Significant changes have occurred within the military in the past 20 years regarding military families on active duty, especially in the move toward professionalization of military family supports. Previously, military family unit support groups were typically led by a commander's spouse who would chair a committee of other spouses, family members, and significant others who would conduct social activities and provide helpful information. While these groups still exist, there are often professional Family Readiness Support staff who provide information, referrals to outside resources, and emergency support when needed. The current military family may look and feel different to what many Americans have become accustomed to in the historic view of the U.S. military. Traditional nuclear families made up of male/female spouses and children remain predominant, but there are growing numbers of same-sex military couples, LGBTQ+ families, remarried and blended families, single service members as parents, children who are homeschooled, and geographically distant relationships by choice and/or necessity. Divorce remains a significant factor of military family life and multiple deployments are often contributing factors to family stress, increased risk, and higher rates of divorce over time.

In terms of military family life, the majority of active-duty children in 2022 were between the ages of 0–11 years, with the largest group being under the age of six years old (40.7%), followed in descending order of 6–11 years (32.9%), 12–18 years (22.5%), and 19–22 years (3.9%). The military family life cycle is typically marked by periods of extended absence of one or more parents due to deployment or extended training away from home, followed by periods of reintegration back into family life. Deployment experiences not marked by serious physical or psychological injuries, traumatic incidents, or other difficulties of military service (including problematic unit cohesion, morale, or leadership), often contribute to an easier reintegration period following a military deployment. If the reintegration into family life is a smooth transition, the family is likely to return to previous levels of family functioning and stability with relative ease. If the reintegration is difficult, however, the family is at risk for heightened stress levels and coping strategies that may not facilitate the return to stability in family life. In these situations, a repeated deployment can be a relief to a family that is not functioning well and not adapting to the stress in healthy ways. The deployment experience is a sacrifice in terms of family life due to the service member's absence from shared family experiences and milestones that make family memories. These losses are significant for families. Every family member copes with them in their own unique, individual ways, and every family

DOI: 10.4324/9781003438229-3

copes with them as a group in a collective way. These long-term absences force family members to manage multiple daily losses in family life while they negotiate and renegotiate their roles and relationships to one another with each separation and reintegration.

> *"The biggest advice I would give to people who begin a long-term relationship with a military service member is to (a) be specific concerning communication with their person, including accepting periods where communication is not available or possible; and (b) identify role expectations within the relationship that place the military couple with shared, co-equal status with one another. While having one person in a dominant role may work for a couple or family in the short term, it often leads to conflict and resentment over time."*
>
> Licensed Clinical Social Worker, U.S. Army Behavioral Health Officer (Uniformed Army Social Workers hold the 73A Military Occupational Specialty)

The deployment experience causes shifts in roles and relationships in families as an at-home spouse or significant other or relative at home is assigned the role of primary caregiver to children, elderly, or other family members in need. This at-home person will move into the dominant role in the family life in terms of running the household, managing finances, making day-to-day financial decisions for the family, obtaining medical treatments for sick or disabled family members, facilitating educational and/or therapeutic supports for children, and managing the physical upkeep of the primary residence if living in a civilian community. The military way of life is one that runs by leadership with tasks and missions completed based on the role of the commander for a team. One of the more challenging aspects of the reintegration period following a military deployment is the renegotiation of roles in family life as military service members often assume that they will return to their previous roles held prior to leaving for a deployment. The at-home spouse, partner, or significant other is likely to experience resistance to a role shift from independence (leadership role in the family) to dependence (stripped of leadership role and responsibilities) especially because that role is now part of that person's identity. Military couples need to negotiate a "new normal" in their relationship to one another and in relation to the other members in the family including children who perceive role changes as confusing. Couples need to find ways to communicate about this process in order to proceed through it with clarity and assurance that both partners agree with a role allocation that allows both partners to be equal contributors in the day-to-day operations and relationships in military families.

In terms of recent numbers, there were more than two million active-duty and reserve service members, with nearly half serving in the Army, the smallest number in the Marine Corps, and almost 2.7 million dependents across the total force. Approximately 50% of military personnel are married, 39% have children, and 6% are single parents (single includes those who are divorced and/or widowed and married includes being re-married); children include dependents aged 20 years or younger and dependents aged 22 years or younger enrolled as full-time students. Currently, 71% of service members reported themselves as White, 17% identified as Black or African American, and 12% reported themselves as multiracial or "race information unavailable." The only information currently reported on ethnicity was that 14% of military personnel identified themselves as Hispanic or Latino. The military collects data regarding race and ethnicity as separate categories, despite the military being racially and ethnically diverse with multiple overlapping identity markers. Military personnel who reported "other/unknown" identities overlapping included 22% of American Indian or Alaska Native personnel, 17% of White personnel, 15% of multiracial personnel, 10% of Native Hawaiian or Other Pacific Islander personnel, 5% of Black or African American personnel, and 4% of Asian personnel (DoD, 2017).

In terms of recent reports on race and ethnicity among active-duty forces, 67% of enlisted personnel identified as White and 19% as Black or African American. Among officer ranks, 77% identified as White and 9% as Black or African American. Although corresponding statistics for the impact of ethnicity on career trajectories was not available, the most recent estimates state that while 18% of active-duty personnel are Hispanic/Latino, only 8% of this population held the rank of an officer (Kamarck, 2019). The DoD reports that the Navy has the most racially diverse active-duty and reserve components; the Marine Corps has the least racially diverse active-duty component; and the Air National Guard has the least racially diverse reserve component in the military. The Marine Corps has the highest percentage of Hispanic/Latino personnel in active duty (21%) with the other service branches reporting 14–15% of personnel being Hispanic/Latino. The reserve components range from 22% identifying as Hispanic/Latino in the Marine Corps Reserves to 6% in the Air Force Reserves (DoD, 2017).

The majority of military personnel identify as male, with 18% female with this cohort increasing annually, with the highest numbers of female service members serving in the Air Force Reserves at 27% (DoD, 2017). In general, the percentage of women in the reserve components (20%) is slightly higher than in the active-duty component at 16% (DoD, 2017). The military occupational specialties reflect traditional civilian female roles as large numbers of female service members are in medical command units, administration roles, and supply units rather than in combat units. In 2016, 25% of active-duty enlisted females worked in administrative careers; 15% were in healthcare; and less than 5% in an occupational specialty in the categories of infantry, gun crews, or seamanship specialists (Office of the Under Secretary of Defense for Personnel and Readiness, 2018).

Military Families in Context

According to recent government reports, there were almost one million (977,954) spouses who were not military personnel themselves across the entire force. The specific age groups for these spouses are as follows: 25 years old or younger (19%); 26–30 years old (23%); 31–35 years old (22%); 36–40 years old (16%); and 41 years or older (20%). The average age of active-duty military spouses was 32 years and the average age for reserve military spouses was 36 years (DoD, 2017). Recent surveys with active-duty spouses reported 61% identified as non-Hispanic White and 38% as Hispanic and/or overlapping racial/ethnic identities. Spouses in the reserve components were reported to have identified as 71% non-Hispanic White and 29% Hispanic and/or overlapping racial/ethnic identities (DoD, 2018). If the survey results are accurate representations for the entire military spousal population, there is more racial/ethnic diversity among active-duty military families than in the reserves. In terms of citizenship among spouses, U.S. Citizenship and Immigration Services (USCIS) reported that in the decade following 2008, approximately 3,000 military spouses became naturalized citizens in ceremonies overseas in more than 35 countries including: Afghanistan, Australia, Chile, China, Germany, India, Norway, Oman, Panama, Philippines, Poland, Tanzania, and Turkey (USCIS, 2017). The most recent survey data reported that 7% of the spouses who responded to the question of citizenship reported not being a U.S. citizen and 6% reported being a U.S. citizen by naturalization. In the same survey, 13% of active-duty spouses reported that English was a second language for them, which is important information to consider when developing policies and programs to accurately meet the needs of military families (National Academies of Sciences, 2019; Defense Manpower Data Center, 2007).

The majority of military spouses are reported to be female: 92% of active-duty spouses and 87% of spouses of the reserves. Although the percentage may appear small in comparison, current estimates report that there are more than 100,000 male spouses married to military service members (DoD, 2017). Married same-sex military couples are eligible for health insurance benefits for reproductive assistance that is not afforded to same-sex military couples who are not married. Despite this availability, many same-sex military couples report not being comfortable self-identifying to the military community due to continued stigma and fears of discrimination resulting from attitudes that have not changed with the change in policies around same-sex marriage. Many same-sex military couples report concerns over active-duty military healthcare due to pervasive negative attitudes from many providers who have limited knowledge and competency to be able to offer affirmative and equitable healthcare.

The military records service member responses regarding gender but not gender identity and one estimate taken from a survey of active-duty service members in 2016 found that 0.6% of service members described themselves as transgender, similar to the percentage of civilian adults identifying this way and less than 1% of respondents declined to answer. According to one estimate, if all the non-responders were transgender, the overall transgender percentage would then be 1.1% (Meadows et al., 2018). The military policy regarding transgender service members has gone through multiple changes from it first being considered a reason for medical disqualification and/or discharge from the military, to the military supporting gender-affirming, medically-necessary transitions in healthcare and treatment for transgender personnel. Policies were drafted regarding the need to meet military standards for the use of gender-appropriate facilities following gender transition. The change in the Administration in 2017 brought about great uncertainty regarding transgender service policies and a delay to these changes with an intention to revert to the previous policy and prohibit transgender military service. These actions met with legal challenges and federal judges were left requesting that a panel of experts prepare revised policy recommendations in response to the uncertainty that continues to remains at this time.

The Active-Duty Military Lifestyle

According to the Department of Defense (2017) data, recruitment strategies for enlisted personnel, who make up approximately 83% of the military, are aimed at recent high school graduates as most new recruits and 40% of the total force are under the age of 25 years. As it is a requirement to have a high school or general equivalency diploma (GED) to enlist in the military, the majority of military personnel (66%) have these as their highest level of education. The remainder have an associate's degree (8%), bachelor's degree (15%), or advanced degree (8%) as their highest level of education (DoD, 2017). As military officers must hold at least a bachelor's degree in order to receive a military commission, they tend to be slightly older on average than enlisted personnel. The minimum age for initial entrance into the military is 17 and the maximum age for entry varies by service branch and according to changing needs within the military. The Marine Corps has traditionally held the youngest maximum age for entry into service (presently 28 years), followed by the Coast Guard (presently 31 years), the Army (presently 35 years), and the remaining three branches of the Navy, Air Force, and Space Force at similar ages (presently all being 39 years). Service members become eligible for retirement after 20 years of service, so individuals who join immediately after high school can retire before the age of 40, enter a second career for another 20 years, and receive retirement benefits from both careers simultaneously.

Military service can expedite the process for non-citizens holding a U.S. Permanent Resident Card (also known as a "green card") who speak, read, and write English fluently to obtain citizenship and more than 125,000 service members became naturalized citizens during the post-9/11 era (U.S. Citizenship and Immigration Services, 2018). Some military occupations require security clearances, however, and because security clearances require citizenship, not all enlisted occupations are open to non-citizens (military officers and warrant officers are required to hold citizenship).

The military requirements for health and fitness are often highest during the developmental stage of early adulthood, which coincides perfectly with the tasks of this stage of forming a new social/group identity while taking on the challenges of adult living. The majority of service members are 18–30 years old and often new to the tasks of independent living that come with adulthood, such as forming a career and taking on roles and responsibilities outside of their families-of-origin. This is a stage of life in which many service members begin thinking about, planning, attempting, and/or forming families and it coincides with primary childbearing ages for women. Military couples or service members who require assistance in starting families sometimes choose to begin the process of reproductive health procedures such as in-vitro fertilization (IVF) to become pregnant and the military supports these procedures if the service member or military couple is married. Many service members will adopt children during active-duty military service, sometimes as a way of starting a new family, and sometimes when a partner already has children or following a divorce and the couple is blending their families together. Given this stage of early adult development, issues of resiliency need to factor in these important life cycle issues, and other relevant tasks that set the contextual background for understanding and enhancing military family well-being.

The Active-Duty Culture of Mobility

There were 1,304,720 active-duty military service members in 2022 according to data reported by Military OneSource with 35% of these members serving in the Army. In the active-duty armed forces, 82% are enlisted personnel (42% of whom are serving at the E1–E4 rank) and the remaining 18% serving in the officer ranks. Geographically speaking, the majority of service members (88% of active-duty and 99% of the reserves) are based in the United States or its territories, and the majority (67%) of active-duty service members are stationed in just 10 states: California, Colorado, Florida, Georgia, Hawaii, North Carolina, South Carolina, Texas, Virginia, and Washington (DoD, 2017). There are more than 40 specific locations designated as being "remote and isolated for morale, welfare, and recreation (MWR) purposes" in the United States (in addition to an equal number outside the United States) that are far from key support services for service members and their families who move with them, including access to quality healthcare and affordable housing.

Orders including a Permanent Change of Station (PCS) usually mean a military move for families and includes military assignments where the service member moves to a new duty station, averaging between two to three years. A military Temporary Duty Yonder (TDY) is an assignment away from one's permanent duty station for training or school and may involve a military family move but can last no longer than 180 days. In some cases, the active-duty service member's family can accompany them for the TDY and would live in a location for just a few months, unless their next set of orders assigns them to the same duty station. Military families may move in situations where a permanent duty station lacks adequate facilities or a medical emergency warrants long-term care, which is common when families stationed overseas discover that a family member needs specialty or long-term care. The long separations of extended deployments are difficult for military families, especially for those with young children and no support networks. In some situations, a service member moves unaccompanied by their family for a PCS move, often overseas, and in such cases military families might make the decision for the military spouse and children to remain at the present duty station or move closer to childhood homes or extended family. Geographic relocations are disruptive to the family's stability and often involve increased levels of anxiety and stress for all family members that has an impact on family functioning as a result. The needs of the military take precedence over the family's needs and families often make great sacrifices when accommodating to those needs and the military lifestyle. Despite social and political changes in most areas of family life in the United States today, the military continues to operate as a male-dominated society rooted in traditional gender stereotypes and a patriarchal system. Needs of dependent family members are typically viewed as less important than the needs of the military and the service member's career within that organization.

At present time, military service members typically move an average of 2–3 years for training missions in new locations, most often in the United States from one state to another. The majority of military families move with the service member and children begin new schools in new states as a result. According to the research, every time a child moves to a new location, children will typically experience significant learning loss in terms of academic achievement and progress attained prior to the move. One study reported that each move during childhood leads to nearly one-half of an academic year lost in terms of educational attainment and that moving three or more times lowered later financial earnings in adulthood by 52% (Ziol-Guest & Kalil, 2014). This study reported that relocating during middle childhood (6–10 years old) was significant in that any move during that period of development was associated with lower earnings, fewer work hours, and less educational attainment later in life. Interestingly, the study also reported that moving in early childhood (0–5 years of age) did not have significant long-term effects in these areas.

In terms of positive child development in active-duty military families, policy development might factor in the risks to school-aged children during the elementary school years. Military families could make decisions about moving based on this information and might choose to remain in one location while the service member moves when the first child in the family begins first grade. This choice would be for families with children in elementary school years to have the service member move to the new location without his or her family, also known as being "unaccompanied by dependents." More research is called for to replicate these findings and offer more data to consider programmatic solutions that would prevent these negative effects across the lifespan of military children. In addition to the educational impact on military youth, there is also the public health implication from associated effects from these moves. These effects may include mental health struggles that include anxiety and depression from feelings that emerge if children are not at the same academic level as their peers and cannot keep pace with academic expectations, or are at a higher academic level compared to peers at a new school. In addition to these, there are also long-term implications that concern the reduced earnings and lower levels of educational achievement attained by a group cohort of military children in the United States.

The average time between PCS moves varies and tends to coincide with a service member's military career. Service members who are unmarried and have no dependents tend to have shorter PCS tours; this is often likely due to being in early stages of their careers (both enlisted and officer ranks) where PCS moves include more training tours which tend to be shorter than operational tours as one progresses in one's career. Service members who have dependents may purposely seek tours that provide their families with more stability when possible although the needs of the military will ultimately take precedence. Among enlisted personnel, those who were more junior (E4 or below) tended to have shorter average PCS tours compared to mid-level (E5–E6) and senior non-commissioned officers (E7–E9) who tended to have the longest average PCS tour lengths. In terms of branch of service, the Marine Corps has the shortest average PCS tours while the Air Force has the longest. The shorter average PCS tour length of the Marine Corps may be due to its greater proportion of first-term enlisted personnel (42%) relative to the other services (which range from 18 to 23%), as more Marines are in the "early career training window" and the average length of time between PCS moves is also related to military occupational specialty (MOS). Enlisted personnel in combat occupations (infantry, artillery, gun crews, seamanship, etc.) had the shortest time between PCS moves, while craft workers (construction, building workers, etc.), and personnel in administrative occupations had the longest. For officers, those in the intelligence and tactical operations areas had the shortest average tours, while scientists, healthcare officers, and administrators had the longest. Service members who averaged less than two years between PCS moves have often reported being less satisfied with the military way of life than those experiencing longer tours, with two years seeming to be the point in time for shifts in satisfaction levels.

Across all the military branches of service, economic concerns dominate the list of most frequently cited PCS problems and include loss or decrease in spouse's income, change in the cost of living, spousal employment, availability of childcare, spousal education, waiting for permanent housing to become available, and temporary lodging expenses. Other reasons for problems during PCS involve timeliness and accuracy of reimbursements, non-reimbursed transportation costs, and costs associated with setting up a new residence. Lower ranking enlisted personnel (grades E1–E3) were more likely than other enlisted personnel to cite problems pertaining to reimbursement and were also more likely to experience "time off at destination to complete move" as a significant problem. Higher ranking enlisted personnel (grades E5–E9) and senior officers (grades O4–O6) were more likely than lower ranking personnel to experience housing-related problems such as waiting for permanent housing to become available, selling or renting a former residence, purchasing/renting and setting up a new residence.

The current military policy of ordering service members to make permanent changes of station every two to three years became more common during the post-9/11 era of military service as PCS moves prior to this time were considerably less frequent. Military spouses earn between 14–24% less during a PCS move than their peers who did not move in that year (Burke & Miller, 2016). This same study found that PCS moves that result in larger reductions in earnings are those that cross state lines and involve older spouses, spouses with young children, and male spouses. Although the contributions of military spouses are acknowledged publicly as being crucial to operational effectiveness by military organizations, policies to improve their situations do not often match this recognition.

Children and adolescents need to adapt to new schools with every move, each time with a new culture, new rules, and even new state laws that govern how they learn, both socially and educationally, within each new academic environment. Health and mental health providers and teachers who interact with children from positions of authority follow state laws and these can be vastly different than other state laws regarding social and political norms. There are states that ban certain discussions and textbooks in education that address heavily debated social topics and have laws that make specific healthcare procedures and treatments illegal while other states welcome and encourage them as parts of healthy development. A child may attend a public school in one of the 19 U.S. states where certain forms of corporal punishment are legal for school administrators to use to discipline children. A child may experience harsh discipline in one school district and then move to a state where this practice may be child abuse and a violation of children's rights. In some school districts, teachers and school staff may not legally use physical restraint on a child even if that child is acting in an unsafe manner. Military children routinely adapt to a different set of rules, laws, expectations, and consequences in new schools and many also manage negative reactions at home if they get into trouble for not adapting well and breaking new rules.

In addition to adjusting to new school environments and new conversations in education and healthcare, many children lose academic skills when they transition to a new school. Moving to a new location during childhood can negatively impact school performance, complex social skills, and prosocial behaviors and these effects accumulate with multiple moves placing children at higher risk than many of their civilian peers. Some children report feeling reluctant to make new friends with each new move because friendships would always come to an end in the physical sense and the loss of these connections is often difficult to bear for a child or teenager already struggling with episodic loss of a military parent. Other military youth have reported relief from knowing that their friendships would come to an end because they never had to resolve any conflicts with peers but learned to "ride it out" until one of them moved away. For these youth, moving to a new location or meeting a new peer group was exciting because it gave them a chance to start over again with a "blank slate" and "re-invent" themselves with each new move. Due to the nature of the military transitions to new locations occurring at different points in every service member's career, children are continuously moving on and off military installations at different rotations than peers. Although the military attempts to have moves occur in the summer months for service members with children, they sometimes do happen in the middle of the school year. Since military families are moving at the pace of the individual service member's career, and not in a group cohort rotation, children are moving in and moving out of one another's lives all the time. For example, a child who moves to a new location and meets a child who has been living there for two years who knows the location and other children well might be perceived by adults as a great person to get to know but the child will quickly realize that that new potential friend will be leaving soon. A new child may keep a distance from potential friends in general as a means of coping with painful feelings around loss, and shy away from opportunities to deepen friendships knowing that they have limited lengths of time. However, a child who has the coping skills to perceive the situation in a different way might decide that although disappointment and hurt are likely to be in the future, they are willing to take that risk for the chance to have a close friend, regardless of how long that friendship lasts. In this manner, the child is resilient and the choice to not focus on the negative outcome sets in motion a cascade of events toward being social and forming new connections despite the brevity and conscious awareness of the finality and pain to come.

Military children go through constant cyclical repetitions of hello and goodbye with friends, neighbors, teachers, coaches, therapists, chaplains, and many more people in their lives but the most significant of these hello and goodbyes happen with their parent who is in the military. The parent who is in military service leaves often and leaves frequently for unexpected work responsibilities, for training missions, and for deployments that can be lengthy tours of duty up to 12–15 months. As a result, military children manage goodbyes from a very early age and form their habits and responses to significant separations based on previous methods that worked for them in the past. Children make behavioral choices daily based on previous coping behaviors that worked for them in difficult situations to help them manage complicated situations and feelings. This process often happens without an awareness that there are multiple choices available to them. For a child to change coping behaviors that have worked for them in the past, such as isolating socially from peers, they need to have support from someone who can explain this process in a language that is developmentally age-appropriate for them. In this way, patterns of behavioral choices can change to ones that are healthy and resilient to manage difficult feelings and situations surrounding loss in the family, with friends, and in their communities of support.

Military Culture, Ethos, and the Warrior Family

The many pieces that make up the military lifestyle are often at odds with one another, as families and the military have competing demands balanced with erratic and constantly changing resources to meet those demands. Many people discuss "bridging the cultural divide" that exists between military and civilian cultures, yet few question if this can ever truly occur. The military exists to defend civilian freedoms that are often taken for granted by civilians that live with the freedom on a daily basis. Critics of the concept of achieving cultural competency raise the issue that lived experiences are so unique that they could never be fully appreciated by individuals who have not lived with the experience themselves. Discussions around cultural humility address being respectfully curious about one's experiences that are different from the person's background to be able to reach a more nuanced understanding of the lived experiences of others from different backgrounds or cultures. The bridge that is firmly entrenched between military and civilian lives cannot be dismantled through an intellectual understanding alone but calls for a genuine humility that can go a long way toward achieving that goal.

Military families live many shared experiences as part of the military culture and lifestyle, one common one being an appreciation for the ever-present threat of war that looms as a possibility at all times. Living with this reality on a daily basis alters many of the views and perceptions about a civilian society that does not live with this experience and vice versa. As a result of this core difference between the cultures, the military family identity is shaped by the reality that a family member who goes on wartime deployment may never return. Deployment cycles bring up the question of who is in and who is out of the family circle quickly and solidifies the family unit as a cohesive system with role exits, role shifts, and role entrances routinely involved in family life. One of the biggest differences in the military lifestyle versus the civilian lifestyle is the experience of the deployment separation. Although not all service members will deploy during their military service careers, they must be "deployable" unless they have special circumstances preventing it and they must be "fit for duty" at all times. Military families vary in structural makeup from service member and civilian spouse; dual-military service career couples; same-sex married military couples; single service members who may never have been married or are divorced, or living with a partner/significant other sometimes sharing childcare or child custody; and multiple other family situations or blended family situations, all united by the readiness to go to war.

Although most active-duty service members are single when they enter the military, they are more likely to be married and to marry at a younger age than their civilian counterparts, have more young children in the household, and there are sharp increases in the numbers of dual-military marriages. The military is an organization with a unique culture that exists and has developed over time to meet the military's needs while meeting the needs of the service members and their families (families are currently the largest cohort in active-duty history). In other times and in previous generations and conflicts, serving in the United States military was something that people did when they were young, sometimes at 17 years old with a parent's permission, and then left as an experience that was part of their young adulthood years. During World War I, World War II, the Korean War, and Vietnam, service members who signed up or were conscripted for military service at a young age were typically unmarried and without children. As in previous generations of military service, military service is for a contracted length of time for serving with the option of renewing that contract if one chooses to do so. While there were always service members who stayed on active duty as a career, the majority of the fighting force seen during wartime served to meet the demands of the military at the time. After their contracts ended, many of these service members left their military service behind, closed the military chapter of their lives, and moved on to new chapters that often included marriage, home ownership, starting businesses, careers, higher education, and having children. All of this was in a linear fashion with each step building upon the next step in a progression where military service was often a patriotic "stepping stone" toward building a rich and fulfilling life.

In the current post-9/11 generation of service member warriors, this was not the typical progression, as the military moved to become an "all-volunteer" fighting force. In the two decades spanning the period following the terrorist attacks in the United States on September 11, 2001, many service members joined straight from high school and remained in service well past the end of their contracts. The biggest difference in terms of social changes was that the current volunteer force began to marry and start families shortly after joining the military. Marriage, children, and a life of domesticity on active duty during wartime was a common occurrence for young service members. While there have always been families on active duty, the volume of young families that faced multiple repeated deployments during wartime was a new chapter in the history of the U.S. military. The majority of young veterans in the post-9/11 wars did not close the chapter of military service after one contract spanning a few years and smoothly transition to life in the civilian world to take advantage of the many benefits available to veterans. This new generation reflected the demands of the military and the seemingly endless wars that taxed the strength of the military and military families with a relentlessness few had seen before that time. Military families experienced instability and chaos on a regular basis, saying goodbye to their family members often, and many endured multiple and lengthy deployments that were often extended in combat zones and other hazardous duty stations for more than 20 years.

The modern military family grew in its identity through these shared unique experiences of deployments, relocations, language, traditions, behaviors, and customs and developed a cultural identity, both inward to the collective military group, and outward to the civilian world as well. The military uses countless words, phrases, and jargon that would be unfamiliar to someone who is not in the military and solidifies membership in the military while also creating a clear distinction of "who is in and who is out" of the group in terms of one's cultural affiliation. Military service members go through a cultural transition of indoctrination when they sign up for military service and attend the initial training or "boot camp" that provides first-hand experience of what military service is all about. This indoctrination into the military culture is fast, intensive, and quickly sets up very clear expectations for what is involved and expected in military service and military culture. Despite a very thorough and intensive indoctrination process into the military for the service members, there still remains lacking an equally-thorough and researched process for transitioning out of the military, and very little of either process for military spouses, children, and significant loved ones.

"Are you military or prior service?" will quickly tell someone if the other person is a part of this group affiliation and quickly cross a hurdle in getting to know someone. The affirmative answer does not automatically create a bond that the media often portrays but starts the ball rolling in terms of whether there might be some comfort zone of familiarity to follow. This is often a lengthier process for family members who may hesitate out of privacy issues or not knowing how such questions will be received one after the next in the series. Questions such as the service member's rank may feel awkward to weave into a first meeting with another family member. In addition to this information, a family member might be curious if the other family experienced deployments, and if so to where, how many, and what the experience was like for the family at home, but hesitate to ask in case this might not be a comfortable topic.

The military culture has countless traditions, rituals, ceremonies, behaviors, expectations and ways for interacting socially that are rooted in generations of repetition over years of patterns of responses. These expectations and shared patterns are there for continuity, clarity, and consistency that are crucial in times of great stress or in chaotic situations. The accumulation of time spent in situations of high stress do not always equate with an increased amount of resistance to that stress and at times the opposite may even occur and weaken the system. Military service members and their families are given a certain level of protection from stress through the sense of stability that comes with being part of a larger social group together with all the rigidity, the rituals, social events, and standards in place for behaviors and appearances that are based upon military ethos.

If you try to define "ethos" you will end up with many definitions, stemming from the time of Aristotle and ancient Greek discussions around issues of moral character, beliefs, and behaviors of an individual, group, or institution. The military ethos reflects the values of the institution and shapes the military identity from the moment a service member enters military life. Service members are required to conform to military regulations for behavior and appearance and to wear the uniform of their branch of service from the moment they enter military service. These behaviors and countless others serve to shape the identity of the service member from a unique individual civilian to one that is part of the military group identity with experiences, beliefs, and values shared by all members. These values and beliefs are part of the military ethos that unifies members as a cohesive group.

In addition to the many traditions and rituals of military life, the military identity is also formed by the environment of the military base, also called an installation, camp, station, port, barracks, or field, depending on the branch of service, and each duty station has its own unique culture within it. Active-duty military families are not required to live in these military environments, however the majority of them choose to do so because it is more cost-effective than living in civilian communities. An important distinction exists between active-duty military families and families of the National Guard and Reserves around the military identity that is formed by the indoctrination into military service. Military families who are not living the "active-duty" military life typically do not experience the culture and the ethos that guide military life found on military installations and the service member in these families is often the only one in the family who understands and lives according to the culture and ethos of the military.

This reality is one of the greatest challenges facing families in the National Guard and Reserves that places them at high risk in terms of psychological resiliency and overall well-being. Military families of the National Guard and Reserves typically have only one member in the military and because of this have a family system that operates according to two sets of cultural identities, two distinct ethos, and at times even two value systems. Resiliency factors for families of the National Guard and Reserve (NG/R) units include the geographic stability that is often found in civilian life and communities filled with neighbors and friends who move much less frequently than in active-duty military communities. Children in these families have the protective factor in place of not having the military requirement of moving to new schools every few years and managing the academic adjustment and sometimes learning loss that accompanies some of these moves. Civilian spouses do not have the same challenges with developing a career trajectory that active-duty military spouses have due to geographic moves. Families of the NG/R units often live in communities with more continuity found in their social support networks over time that serves as a protective buffer in times of stress.

Children and families in the NG/R often have different experiences in terms of conflict resolution over long-term relationships and managing relationship distress in community social networks. Due to the constant geographic relocations that are currently present in active-duty military service every 2–3 years, families who are constantly moving need only to wait until a new move to see a conflict with a friend or neighbor disappear entirely. When conflicts arise, active-duty families do not need to resolve or manage feelings of discomfort in social relationships outside of the family unit. Due to the constant moving and the behavioral expectations in active-duty families, there is a tendency to let conflicts outside of the family go unresolved. Children growing up in cultures where conflicts are tolerated and unresolved because of the brevity of the social relationships (with friends, peers, coaches, teachers, and neighbors) do not get to practice and develop valuable skills for managing relationship dilemmas. Social supports are different for NG/R families compared to active-duty military families in terms of the continuity of relationships that require resolving conflicts when they arise or risk losing them entirely. In addition to this is often the presence of extended family networks that often provide a safety net and can buffer the effects of stress when a family needs it. While active-duty families receive much support from the military organization, they are isolated geographically from their families-of-origin and consistent social support networks, and families of the NG/R may lack unit-based support but be surrounded by generations of extended family supports.

Despite the differences, all military families share the military experience of deployments (actual or looming), as well as the identity, ethos, and values that are crucial aspects to understanding the multiple influences that motivate family choices, both daily and in long-term planning. If you ask military-connected individuals to list some of the core values that guide their everyday life, you will likely get an answer without much hesitation. Values such as honor, integrity, respect, duty to country, honesty, hard work, loyalty, and family may be among those listed in rapid-fire and sometimes even having sub-sections within those values described. Values make up a guiding compass for service members and military families alike and are extremely helpful in talking about social identity and how the intersection of values, identity, and behavior impact daily life. Discussions around values need to be included when working with veterans, service members, military couples experiencing marital distress, or military-connected families in crisis. It is easy for values to be lost in the midst of a crisis or stressful situation, but they are crucial influences that shape our perceptions and responses to the situation. Identifying and living by one's values provides a stabilizing force in finding solutions to manage stressful situations. The influence of one's value system can assist in choosing behavioral responses that are adaptive, healthy, and resilient in nature. Individuals and families who are highly resilient tend to make a quick and thorough assessment of a stressful situation and accept that certain aspects of it cannot be changed or modified. Once the areas that can be influenced or changed are identified, resilient responses are able to emerge that are in line with that family's value system and make sense to all individual family members.

The military culture consists of a shared language that is familiar to service members and their families within military environments and a language not often used outside of these environments. The reason the language is insular to the military is due in part to the fact that very few individuals in the civilian world are familiar with common terms used in military life. Many military family members will explain that while it may be easy to translate these terms, it is easier not to use them in the presence of civilians who are unfamiliar with them. For example, military families routinely use the term "PCS" which translates into "Permanent Change of Station," as a verb in discussions around geographic relocations. In conversations with civilians, neither the acronym not the translation of it would tend to suffice as a definition to a non-military person who would need yet a third definition along the lines of "We're moving to a new base installation." The term "installation" would then need to be defined and include that the service member was ordered to a different military base in a different location in a different state or country. If the family was to live off base, this would need to be included in the explanation as well and there would likely be questions about the choice or reasons for off-base housing versus base housing. If a military family member were telling another military family member, it would be much faster with fewer explanations needed, as in "We're PCS'ing to Drum in July." The statement would carry with it a host of information on the history of the base in terms of the base's culture, the work that is generally done there, and the grapevine of stories shared between service members and military families who have lived and worked there previously. In the event that someone was unfamiliar with these stories and the legacy of a base's culture, someone would eventually intervene to offer stories that they have heard or experienced themselves.

The military family that lives on a military base is expected to uphold the many customs and standards of behavior that the service member must uphold. For example, driving on base is very slow with speed limits tending to be not more than 20 mph and enforced by military police to ensure safety and security on the base. In the military environment, there are multiple traditions, ceremonies, and events that occur every day and unify all members in that community with the respect and seriousness attributed to them. The traditions of reveille and retreat, the raising and lowering of the American flag, is accompanied by bugle music that signals the start and end of the workday while also serving to reinforce the core values of the military. Service members who are outdoors will stop whatever they are doing, turn toward the flag, stand at attention, and salute the flag. If family members are present outdoors at these times, they are expected to stop what they are doing as well and if driving to stop the vehicle until this tradition is concluded. The playing of "Taps" occurs every evening on military bases to both honor fallen service members and signal the beginning of quiet hours. Social events are another tradition that is an expectation but not a requirement in military family life that foster military identity and the group cohesiveness. Career promotions, change of command ceremonies, military balls, and family picnics provide immediate social support and friendship to the community. The lifestyle of the military culture is constantly welcoming new members and saying goodbye to others and military events help to build the "esprit de corps" and strengthen a sense of belonging to the military community (Scott, Whitworth, & Herzog, 2017). The sense of belonging that develops and strengthens throughout military service (assisted by the ethos, lifestyle, and shared cultural identity) is what is often responsible for a deeply experienced, acute sense of loss at it being missing once service members and military families transition out of military service. Many individuals with prior military service end up working for the military as civilian government contractors and in careers that share this sense of camaraderie, such as often found among first responders. Active-duty military spouses and children often report surprise and disappointment that civilian friendships are so difficult to forge outside of the military and that civilian peers or neighbors keep their distance when family members look to them for support. Social experiences like these following active-duty military service often leave family members longing for this aspect of military life where friendships and social connections were easier (and possible) to make. Individual family members who experience this difficulty are often left feeling isolated in their new civilian community and at risk for depression as a result, especially if they personalize situations and blame themselves for any failed attempts at forming new relationships with their civilian peers. While the military does an excellent job at indoctrinating service members and their families into the military community, they often disappoint at the other end of military service, when all family members would benefit from education and awareness that these are universal experiences.

Military families live in multiple locations, states, and countries and installations are under federal jurisdiction and federal land geographically. Due to the high mobility and living in federal areas, military children (and sometimes military spouses as well) will have difficulty stating where they are from when civilians ask this question. Federal rules apply legally and necessary items such as food and clothing that is purchased within a military installation are exempt from state taxes which significantly lower the costs of living while on active duty. For this reason, many military retirees and family members will drive great distances to go shopping on a military base to purchase household items. Alcohol is the only mood-altering psychoactive substance that is allowed on active-duty installations as it is the only one that is legal in all states. The recent legalization of cannabis in many states is not legal in all states and due to this, it is illegal for service members as well as military family members to possess marijuana on a military base even if they are not using the substance. The possession of marijuana on base is illegal and treated as such, even if the base in located in a state that has legalized its use. This becomes complicated for adolescents who often attend high school in civilian communities off base and interact with other teenagers who live with the substance being legal for adults in their communities. The fact that it is still illegal to possess or use marijuana until an adolescent reaches 21 years old is often lost on adolescents drawn to experiment with alcohol or other substances.

Active-duty military families live in communities that require that the needs and demands of the military and the military parent take priority over family life. Military spouses and children on active-duty bases are required to adhere to a strict set of behaviors for both inside the family and outside in the community. Although military family members do not fall under the military itself, and as such are not required to abide by the same rules that govern behavior, they are also not encouraged to behave in public with behaviors that place the military service member at risk by association. A military service member is expected to pay attention to their family to maintain family stability and predictability for everyone. A military commander will be informed of situations that involve the military police responding to military families in crisis on base or who are getting into trouble for conduct that is not according to the military codes or rules for security on the base. Examples of this include situations of domestic abuse, interpersonal violence, having affairs outside of a marriage, drunk or disorderly conduct, getting into fights, or possessing illegal substances including marijuana. Although military family members have certain freedoms that military service members do not possess, such as the freedom of speech, there are expectations, both said and unsaid, regarding behavior and behavioral standards for family members as well as for service members. Military family members are civilians and as such allowed to express their opinions and views about politics, wars, and the military chain of command without direct impact to themselves. There is an indirect impact, however, if such speech is seen as creating a negative climate in the military community and/or threatens the comradery and unit cohesion that the military organization strives to maintain. Military service members exist within a positive climate regarding the military and negative behaviors by family members will likely reflect negatively on the service member. It is expected that service members, and their families, will refrain from behaviors that threaten that positive climate and service members may have to explain public speech, behaviors, or even social media posts that appear as overly negative or divisive in nature.

Military Family Virtues

In addition to the shared set of core values among military service members, and many families by association, there is also a shared set of virtues present that fill in the background context of military life and serve to guide and shape daily behaviors. The virtues of courage, boldness, strength, and stamina are easily recognizable to non-military civilians but other, more nuanced ones, that guide perspectives and may not be as easily identified, concern issues of ethics and morality (Exum, Coll, & Weiss, 2011). The authors summarize previous works on the virtues of peacefulness, restraint, and obedience that operate to guide military leadership in relation to wartime and the many moral obligations involved in military service. The U.S. military does not have one set of ethical standards for behavior but has many codes for conduct that embody the values and virtues of military culture. The two that tend to exert the most influence over military family life include the Chain of Command and the Uniform Code of Military Justice, especially for active-duty families living on military bases. These codes of conduct cross over into military family life and guide daily behaviors as well as define the consequences of not doing so. Among the many virtues found in military culture and ethos, the guidance that these codes offer gives a sense of stability in times of confusion or uncertainty in the belief that every situation has a response that is appropriate. In terms of resiliency, the most effective response is often the one that follows a clear path based on one's values for proceeding through situations that can otherwise become chaotic or influenced by one's emotions. An example of this virtue is illustrated in one study with military spouses that found that being task-oriented, rather than emotion-oriented, in terms of problem-solving was an adaptive coping strategy that led to increased levels of resiliency and overall well-being (Wang et al., 2018).

Task completion is generally associated with feelings of satisfaction and in situations needing solutions, distraction from one's feelings can be very effective. Military family life and military service are competing institutions and highly demanding in that they both require complete dedication, commitment, and attention to completing tasks. The military/warrior society is one that is mission-driven and requires maximum performance in terms of fitness, strength, and heightened achievement levels that can be developed and thrive in young adulthood. There is a mandatory age for retirement in the military based on a service member's years in service and rank attained. Mandatory retirement is unique to the military and creates an entire culture of young adults without a generation of older mentors, aging parents, and grandparents to offer advice and wisdom based on life lessons learned. It also creates a gap for military families who have no extended support networks for socializing, dinners together, babysitting, and celebrations or holidays spent together.

The social characteristics of the military culture, including the intersection of this culture and the military family living in the "social fortress" of the active-duty military, are described in great detail in previous texts of Wertsch (1991) and Hall (2016) and many of these are listed in Figure 1.1. The many characteristics listed here are compiled from these significant contributions that present great understanding and appreciation of the experience of growing up in an active-duty military family. In recent years, the Military Child Education Coalition disseminated significant education and training to civilian community providers who worked with military children to support their inherent strengths and foster resiliency during the wars in Iraq and Afghanistan. Some of the common reasons that service members join the military were included in these trainings to describe the motivation and dedication seen in military members and their families to civilian teachers, counselors, and school administrators. Reasons included a family history, tradition, and legacy of being in the military; benefits to joining including financial stability; peer groups and the identity as a warrior; a sense of belonging to something bigger than their own worlds; and sometimes to escape their homes and seek out new adventures as adults separate from their birth families. The military life comes with a pattern of collectively shared experiences. These include the following: frequent separations and reunions; regular geographic relocations; the demands of the military taking priority over family life; a sense of rigidity, regimentation, and conformity to a set of rules and time honored traditions; early retirement from a military career with financial stability; an ever-present background threat of danger and death; feelings of detachment from mainstream America; a system that meets the family's needs; travel and adventure constantly and routinely; and social ties and effects of the service member's position on family behaviors and lifestyle choices (Hall, 2016).

The military functions best due to the hierarchical model where every service member follows orders of a leader above them all the way up the chain of command to the Commander-in-Chief, the President of the United States. Leadership is encouraged throughout all levels in this chain of individuals who are parts of a team that is part of a larger group of teams working in tandem with one another for maximum efficiency. The military's group within group model works from a collectivist perspective that views the success of the group as more important than any one individual member within that group. This group-focused way of life is very different than the American ideal of individualism that believes in the power of the individual to succeed based on reaching whatever goals one sets for self or family. In terms of military missions, an individual focus would fail to succeed and would even be dangerous to the safety and stability of everyone in the group, and the group as a whole. It has been noted that one of the great paradoxes of the military is that its members, the self-appointed guardians of American democratic values, do not live in a democracy themselves (Wertsch, 1991).

There is a sense of isolation and alienation from the civilian world for military service members and their families, especially those living on active-duty bases, with an expectation that certain information does not lend itself to easily being shared outside that community. The distinct characteristics of the civilian culture of the United States include a focus on individuality, individual achievement, personal freedom, and fluid social mobility, all of which are in opposition to the precepts of the military culture (Exum, Coll, & Weiss, 2011). There is an inward focus in the military due to the hierarchical class structure and outward to the civilian world due to the differences. The military culture's strict social structure emphasizes the mission and group solidarity in pursuit of that mission with social status being very clear in the military and earned meritoriously by one's rank which sets pay scales and determines military housing. Military work ethics take priority and set standards for the work of the mission at hand above all else. These differences and alienation exist for military spouses and children as

Social Characteristics of The Fortress

- Authoritarian Structure
- Isolation & Alienation
- Class System
- Parent Absence
- Eternal Youth
- Importance of Mission
- Prepared for Disaster

Warrior Society: Characteristics

- Frequent Separations & Reunions
- Regular Geographic Relocations (PCS)
- "Mission Always Comes First"
- Rigidity, Regimentation, Conformity
- Early Retirement from Military Career
- Background Threat of Death during Missions
- Feelings of Detachment from Mainstream America
- System Meets the Family's Needs
- Travel & Adventure
- Social Effects of Rank on Family

Psychological Characteristics of The Fortress

- Secrecy: Keeping work & family separate; not talking about what goes on at work when home
- Stoicism: Keeping the appearance of stability
- Denial: Need to keep all feelings & fears underground, not expressed or shared
- Shame: For feelings of weakness, guilty for feeling fear, vulnerability of despair, or for needing help.

Figure 1.1 Social characteristics of the fortress, warrior society: characteristics, and psychological characteristics of the fortress

well due to the vast gap between the military and civilian cultures that has yet to be fully bridged, embraced, or understood. Potential family dynamics that can arise in military families to manage conflicts include arguments prior to military-related separations or deployments as a way to disengage from the painful feelings of upcoming separation and loss. In addition to separations, military families may find that it is easier to tolerate the upheaval, chaos, and role confusions of the deployment cycle with the idea that it is a temporary stage and feelings will get resolved once the service member leaves or returns from a deployment. Parents may cope with family upheavals by disengaging emotionally through alcohol, working, or other means of distancing from family life; and military children may become nervous in anticipation of a military parent returning rather than leaving (Hall, 2016).

Civilian Warriors Called to Active Duty

The National Guard and Reserve components of the military accounted for approximately one-half of the total fighting force of the post-9/11 wars yet almost none of these families lived on military bases. Historically, following the conflict in Vietnam, the United States ended the policy of conscription into military service. The Abrams Doctrine formally ended the system of involuntarily drafting young men into war in 1973, however despite the end of conscription, all young men are still required to register with the Armed Services on their 18th birthday in the United States. Despite the U.S. military's inclusion of women into combat roles, these women volunteered for these roles and if conscription were to be practiced again, the military has stated that they would not conscript women into combat roles. The courts have repeatedly deferred to Congressional authority regarding military personnel law and policy related to national security interests. In a case titled "*Rostker v. Goldberg*," [453 U.S. 57 (1981)], the U.S. Supreme Court determined that it was "not unconstitutional" to require only men to register for the draft, and that Congress was entitled, in the exercise of its Constitutional powers, to focus on the question of "military need rather than equity." In this way, the military is not subject to the same employment standards as civilian society and continues in many ways to be a patriarchal institution steeped in traditions that have been in place for hundreds of years.

The historical perspective is necessary to describe the context and the setting in which the military family emerged during the rising volunteer force of peacetime following the Vietnam era. In tandem with the Abrams Doctrine and end of conscription following Vietnam, a significant shift in policy regarding National Guard units placed them in ready position to fill the gap that conscription had filled should war ever break out again. As our history with war seemed a distant past for nearly 30 years of relative peacetime, shortly following the attacks on 9/11, National Guard troops were called to abide by their oath and were mobilized to war. The definition of a military family suddenly included civilian families with no previous experience of living an active-duty military lifestyle and scarce supports in place for them. Most family members of the National Guard and Reserve units had never stepped foot inside a military base or installation and had never seen their military family member hold or carry a weapon, even those whose family member held an occupational specialty in the Infantry. National Guard/Reserve service members were called on to serve repeated and lengthy combat deployments, sometimes lasting 12–15 months, without the support structure in place of the active-duty military for these families.

Service members from the NG/R returned from combat deployments to civilian jobs and civilian lives as if they had been on extended work trips. These military families lived on both sides of a cultural divide sometimes knowing nothing about the military side and with virtually no one supporting them through the experience. Family Readiness Groups sprouted up that were voluntarily run by other family members, sometimes siblings, who also knew very little about the military organization, lifestyle, culture, values, virtues, codes for conduct, norms for social behavior, and little about the effect of rank structure on families. Typically, one or two family members were employed by Military One Source as civilian contractors to offer assistance and referrals for support for thousands of families. There was no formal support in civilian communities since for the most part civilians were not being impacted by the wars, often didn't follow media coverage, and had little-to-no understanding of international current events, nor the military's role in them. For all intents and purposes, families of Guard and Reserve service members were left on their own to go through the extremely stressful experience of sending a family member into combat during wartime. The National Guard had been kept out of going to war during Vietnam in order to protect national interests at home and to serve in situations of national and state emergencies, floods, hurricane relief, and anything else that needed large-scale responses to risks of national security. The majority of the National Guard service members were working one weekend per month and two weeks in the summer for training exercises, serving mostly under the governor of the state in which they resided. These service members were informally termed "Weekend Warriors" and took the sworn oath to defend the Constitution against all enemies, foreign and domestic, should they be needed to go to war, although many had never done so, and many families never expected that they would do so. These service members were not living within military units on military bases, had none of the supports in place of active-duty life, yet deployed into combat roles repeatedly for up to 20 years. In between deployments, these Weekend Warriors trained with their units one weekend per month (returning home at night) and two weeks in the summer during annual trainings. The total time these units spent together on active duty was an approximate total of about one month per year.

Military Cultural Competency and Cultural Humility

The concept of achieving cultural competency in the helping professions has focused on practitioners gaining knowledge, language, and skills to better treat individuals from cultural backgrounds different from their own. As many healthcare providers are from the dominant culture in power, with the privilege of being able to afford the highest levels of education attainable, the consequence of increasing the academic knowledge base concerning non-dominant cultures has sometimes paradoxically created less understanding for lived experiences as a result. Providers who acquire knowledge through courses and research about a culture can actually reinforce the dominant perspective if information used to make treatment plans does not happen without the individual's crucial input. The unforeseen and widely unintended consequence of cultural competency training is that providers have sometimes become less effective with increased knowledge about non-dominant cultures. For example, providers who believe they know about a client's culture can quickly make assumptions about behaviors or symptoms and fail to ask important questions or solicit input from their clients or patients. In this counterintuitive chain of events, clients do not have the opportunity to tell their stories from their perspectives, the role of practitioner-as-expert becomes solidified, and the power imbalance is further entrenched and reinforced systemically as a result.

Cultural humility, on the other hand, is understood as holding an interpersonal perspective that is other-oriented rather than self-focused on the provider and his or her acquisition of knowledge and skills (Hook et al., 2013). Practitioners who employ cultural humility do not use knowledge or skills learned to elevate themselves to the role of expert about a culture but rather, inquire about the lived experiences and perspectives of their clients, with a genuine curiosity that places the client in the role of the expert. The incorporation of cultural humility in mental health treatment allows for collaborative problem solving that is strengths-based and does not allow for superiority to result that diminishes any individual or culture in the process.

In working with military, cultural competency trainings without the lens of cultural humility to factor in the diversity of lived experiences and intersecting identities keeps the role of practitioner-as-expert in place. The Veterans Health Administration is the largest healthcare organization that treats veterans and reflects the uniformity of the military organization even though its clients are no longer in the military. Meetings are often scheduled in military time and the value of a hierarchical organizational structure is evident from the minute you step in the doors and often during interactions you have with treatment providers while there. The predominant use of the medical model prevails and the hierarchical model of treatment is based on the practitioner-as-expert built into the systemic culture. Cultural competency trainings for healthcare providers working with military-connected communities often focus around the areas of knowledge, language, and skills. Topics include the endless list of the acronyms used in the military; the rank and military grade structure; understanding the beliefs and assumptions, both spoken and unspoken, held about the military lifestyle; the fears, goals, and complications of living with long and frequent absences inherent in military family life; understanding the frequent relocations and expectations for moving to undesirable places every few years; and gaining a clear understanding of the subtle lifestyle changes that families endure with all of these relocations and separations.

Multicultural competency and cultural humility combined involve becoming aware of the impact of our behavior, values, biases, preconceived notions, and personal limitations so that we may understand the worldviews of culturally diverse individuals without negative judgment. It requires that we actively develop and practice appropriate, relevant, and sensitive strategies in working with culturally diverse clients (Hall, 2016). Every culture has characteristics that are unique to the identity of that group and the military is a culture that has a long history of its identity, shared traits, and characteristics. There is a common language and code for manners, a shared dress code, shared expectations for behavior, shared belief systems, shared ideas about family life, as well as shared rituals and traditions. Despite all of these shared experiences, individuals have their own unique perspectives on these experiences (see Figure 1.2).

Despite the military being designed with teams working together in a collective manner to achieve its goals, the merits of the individual service member working on those teams is encouraged so that they can be promoted to the next rank and assume a leadership role in the chain of command. The military is often referred to as a pure meritocracy because the skills and abilities of service members are valued, celebrated, and rewarded. The concept of the military being a pure meritocracy has been challenged by the presence of a reported glass ceiling for women and minority groups for promotion to the highest ranks. The history of institutionalized racism continues to affect African American, Black,

Competency	Humility
1. Self-Focused	1. Other-Focused
2. Practitioner as Expert	2. Client as Expert
3. Empowers Practitioner	3. Empowers Client
4. Hierarchical Treatment Diminishes Client	4. Collaborative Problem-Solving Treatment
5. Power/Superiority Results	5. Strength-Based Results

Figure 1.2 Cultural competency vs. cultural humility

Latino, and Indigenous service members and other minority groups who are denied leadership roles at the highest levels and debunks the myth of the military meritocracy. Although the military is culturally diverse and represents a system of promotion based on one's abilities, it continues to promote career advancement of predominantly White male service members to the highest ranks and stems that advancement for other groups based on race, ethnicity, gender, and sexual identity/orientation.

The now debunked and outdated belief that the military is a pure meritocracy parallels another challenge highlighting the great divide between military and civilian ways of life in the difference in the work ethic. The military culture is one in which individuals may be tasked and expected to work long hours if a mission needs to be completed. Living with this type of a work ethic often makes it difficult to understand a work ethic that does not involve such expectations and in certain situations, some civilians may be viewed as lazy, or selfish and unmotivated, and not a team player. There is often also difficulty understanding some civilian leisure activities that have no secondary gain and can be thought of as wasting precious time and the notion of self-care can be seen as self-indulgent or self-centered. At times, some civilians may be viewed as lacking motivation in terms of physical fitness, mental fitness, adaptability to change, and family wellness and well-being as a critical part of a cohesive, closely-knit, and functioning team. There are also challenges for military service members and their families in understanding non-military individuals and families and is most noticeably evident in different perceptions about the civilian sense of individualism and focus on self that permeates many aspects of life. These views also influence values, attitudes, and behaviors regarding choices in career, work ethics, and family values including parenting styles. There are various opinions about civilians who are living civilian lives in a cultural context that affords multiple levels of freedoms that are often seen as being taken for granted. This can be a source of pride and it can also be a source of frustration for some military service members who may perceive it as being under-valued or under-appreciated when it is witnessed through social interactions and experiences in civilian life.

Culture, Climate, and the Collectivist Perspective

Organizational climate refers to the perception and attitudes of service members as they interact with their peers, subordinates, and leaders. Climate can significantly influence many critical outcomes such as readiness, performance, morale, motivation, mutual respect, and discipline. Therefore, it's essential that units are committed to promoting healthy, positive climates and all members are expected to be responsible for contributing to that positive climate. Military leaders are expected to not only create a positive climate, but also to maintain that climate, by setting an example for behaviors of doing what is right at all times in all circumstances. The importance of trust is crucial to creating a positive climate both in the vertical axis up and down the chain-of-command and in a horizontal axis between peers within units. Military leaders earn the trust of their team when they lead by example and demonstrate good character, competence, and commitment to the team and the team's missions.

There is a distinction in the military between climate and culture and this is important because it allows service members to know what they have influence over and what they do not. When viewed as an iceberg, climate is what is seen above the water line, and refers to what can be observed, together with the day-to-day perceptions and feelings, and affects the motivation and trust of individuals. Climate can be difficult to change but when it does, change can happen quickly, and is shaped by an organization's direct leaders. Culture, on the other hand, is below the water line and made up of deeply embedded beliefs and customs that are long-standing and difficult to change.

Culture consists of a shared set of beliefs, values, norms, and symbols that unite a group and characterize the larger institution over time. Culture evolves slowly and is deeply rooted in long-held beliefs that are passed down from one generation to the next. Military culture can be viewed on a daily basis through the many regulations, policies, doctrine, customs, traditions, songs, and the warrior ethos. In the military culture, the values of trust, military expertise, service, stewardship, and esprit de corps are held in high regard for their influence on daily living. Leadership in the military relies on this culture and reminds members that they are part of something bigger than themselves, with responsibilities based on being a point in time in history. Organized militaries have existed for centuries and the cultural perspective of most present-day military organizations is that they will exist into the future as well to defend the beliefs and freedoms of the larger civilian society. Military members perceive that their contributions to the military are their contributions to their civilian society and see their group as part of an organization that is rooted in the past and will exist into the future. This historical perspective offers members a sense of belonging to a greater experience than their own lives, which are short in comparison to thousands of years of shared collective experiences defending civilian society.

Climate is how members think and feel about their community and is shaped by shared perceptions, attitudes, and behaviors about day-to-day life. The collective daily living experiences influence individual motivation for how things are done and trust in one's peer networks and leaders. Climate tends to be a short-term experience that changes as people enter and exit roles making it much easier to change climate than it is to change culture. Military organizational climate influences service members in terms of their individual and group motivation, job satisfaction, morale, cohesion, commitment, initiative, trust, and general overall performance. Military organizations aim to be "high-performing organizations" as the alternative to this can mean failure and massive loss of life as a result. In order to prevent this from happening, military organizations state that they require what is considered a "positive command climate" to be successful in achieving their goals. The reason why a positive climate is so important to the military, and to any high-performing organization, is that the success of the organization is the ultimate goal and a negative organizational climate is a major obstacle to success. Organizations with negative climates are more likely to struggle to adapt to changing environments because they do not work well as a team together, have increased disciplinary issues, fail to meet expectations for performance, and are less likely to achieve their overall aims and stated goals.

The idea of the positive command climate extends to the military family as well because service member morale and occupational performance are vulnerable to influences in one's home life. As a result, the organization strives to sustain positive morale in military family life. In the ecological theory of organizations, the military family is a micro-system that influences the service member who influences the wider military community. The ultimate success of the organization as a whole relies on circles of influence that get wider and wider and exert influence on one another in the process. The presence of a negative family climate for any individual service member has the potential to place the entire organization at risk for failure as a result. Active-duty military families possess multiple protective factors by living in a community that provides for the necessities of life. Reduced costs for early childhood day care for children, availability of affordable housing, free education, and other social supports are present on military bases. These supports are helpful in managing the demands of the military lifestyle that impact a family's adaptation to stress. There are constant challenges present in the military lifestyle that impact family dynamics and require routine adaptations to change that far exceed those experienced in most civilian families. In addition to the multiple adaptations required as a result of the regular geographic relocations and changes in schools and communities, there are also multiple adaptations to shifting roles and relationships in the family system that are much more complex and dynamic in nature. The military family endures role shifts and changes in daily routines and patterns in the family system at such a regular occurrence in life that few other systems could sustain without breaking down. The fact that military families not only survive, but often thrive, in the midst of these challenges and become stronger is a result of an entire organization needing them to do so by addressing issues that arise immediately and with a sense of urgency. Resiliency emerges in military families due to the fact that challenges are managed and failure is not an option for a family in crisis.

There are clear benefits that come with the collectivist perspective that is part of the military organizational context including a strong cultural affiliation and ties to the military, its worldview and perspectives on strength, health, and well-being of its members. The intersection of military culture with other significant cultural influences such as race, ethnicity, gender, and sexual orientation helps to better understand the nature and complexity of military family life. Some of the shared experiences of military family life include the regular absence of the service member from family life and missing significant family milestones including birthdays, holidays, anniversaries, sporting events, and graduation ceremonies. In addition to routine absences of the service member from family life, these absences are often unpredictable, sudden, and of varying lengths and levels of risk involved. Military family members adapt to not knowing if the military service member will be present or not as a routine part of family life. In civilian families, the repeated absence of a parental figure would have different meanings attributed to the absences that would influence the family's overall adaptation to the stress of the situation. In military families, however, the episodic loss of the military parent to work, or lengthy deployment situations, is an experience that is normative in the community. Although every child is unique, sharing collective experiences that are not traumatic or overly negative generally serves as a protective factor in being able to adapt to stress in resilient ways. Active-duty military children witness other military children and families experience regular separations and disruptions in their daily lives and attachments with their parents. For families living on bases with other families, this collective group experience helps to make losses and crises more manageable as the lifestyle is normative for everyone on a military base. Military families of National Guard and Reserve components do not have the active-duty collective experiences, however, and manage the crises of military-related family separations from the civilian context. Families in the reserve components are often at higher risk in terms of resiliency to the stress of deployment separations because the experience is often not one that is shared with anyone in their communities. The meaning that is attached to the stressful situation of a military deployment is one of isolation and more likely to be experienced as a crisis in the family's adaptation to the stress as a result.

Resilience in the military context depends on being part of a much larger group effort also known as the mission of the organization that is larger than the self and using military force in teams where survival depends on working together. The military organization is a machine because all of the parts rely on each other to work and the use of the term "weak link" is associated with being the part that could be responsible for its failure. If any part of the organization is not capable in their role, the entire mission may be at risk as a result. Despite the detailed focus on training military service members, the organization remains at risk if families are not resilient. As the next generation of warrior families emerges, the organization is capable of meeting the needs of the military family through the lessons learned from the previous two decades of wartime military service.

Case Example

A few days before Thanksgiving, a military spouse was on a three-hour layover after midnight in the LAX airport after the first leg of a journey to visit her family with a toddler in tow. Feeling exhausted, she went to sit in an area with other children running around so her daughter could play with them and she could get a few minutes to check emails without needing to entertain her. There were other families who seemed to have had their flights significantly delayed or cancelled due to weather storms that had been going on around Los Angeles that night creating many weary travellers all stuck together in a collective sense of shared misery and fatigue.

As she was about to sit down, the spouse saw a young mother with three small children by herself attempting to not only entertain a 2-year-old and a 4-year-old, but simultaneously changing the diaper of an infant in tow. She had created a makeshift changing station as a "workaround" for not having a bathroom nearby and it was clear that she could never bring all of her luggage, and her children, to a far-off bathroom and still maintain possession of her seats in the gate area. She unfolded a large diaper-changing pad near the window and was negotiating with both a crying baby and her other children's wants and needs at the same time. The baby was stretched out resisting the mother's attempts to change the diaper and get a pajama onesie onto her and the 3-year-old was making repeated attempts to run away from them to pull his older sister's hair for fun and get out some pent-up energy he had stored up from the last plane ride.

The spouse went over to see if she could help the mom whom she felt empathy for since she was on her own as well and managing three children to her one so knew instantly that she had it much easier by sheer magnitude alone. She immediately created a wider, group-focused game of "catch me if you can" that she was playing anyway without rules to it with her daughter who joined in as well so it was a "win-win" situation for everyone. The second, younger mother finished diaper changing and pajama dressing her baby and got up to join the play. As she was rocking her baby to sleep with one arm and catching her escaping toddler with the other, she quickly sized up the situation, which she was apparently very good at doing, from a combination of experience and necessity. She saw that the spouse was there: without a partner, with a child, stranded at an airport in the middle of the night, going to visit family for the holidays, and had jumped in to help her when no one else who was partnered at the gate area had done.

She didn't hesitate and asked immediately: "Are you military?" The spouse didn't have an answer, partly because she was exhausted but mostly because she didn't know the correct answer to the question. Clearly this was a "yes" or "no" type of question and in her fatigued state, she hesitated and chose "no" for her answer. She was immediately caught off guard by this young woman, who by all appearances had more wits about her than she did despite her much younger age, and conveyed a sense of complete competence in the midst of chaos. She sensed the older spouse's hesitation and asked again yet in a different way that was instantly more disarming and invited an explanation rather than demanded an answer: "Oh, it's just that you seem military to me." The spouse felt compelled to explain somehow since the woman with three tired children tugging at her had opened a door with warmth and compassion in her tone of voice despite her stressful situation: "Well, my husband is in the military, but I'm not." The younger woman's smile grew wider but not in a condescending or critical manner but rather one that offered support and as she maintained direct eye contact, she simply stated, "I knew it." The older spouse was confused again. She knew what exactly and how did the answer give her any degree of insight or information into her life? The spouse hadn't told her anything personal to that point so she decided to explain: "Well, my husband is in the Navy Reserves and is now deployed to the Middle East for a year." The older spouse's explanation of the details of her husband's service didn't change the younger woman's opinion that she had arrived at by then: that the older spouse had arrived at by then that she was a military spouse and she told the woman that her husband was on a deployment as well. She smiled warmly and then stated as an unquestionable fact: "Chica, if your husband is military, then you ... are ... military."

2 Resiliency in the Military Family

The Markers of Resiliency

What makes military families able to adapt to the constant levels of stress involved in the military family's lifestyle? Some military family members report that staying focused on tasks and goal achievement during times of stress, rather than on emotions, is adaptive and prevents family members from falling into depressive states. In addition to certain individual baseline temperaments being less reactive and more adaptable to stress, patterns of behaviors in families such as direct communication and open emotional expression have been shown to increase resiliency. There are certain features for individuals and families that are hallmarks for resiliency that fall into internal beliefs and external behaviors. Internal beliefs include our views, perspectives on health and wellness, opinions about ourselves, others, and perceptions of safety in the world. The ways in which we think about our problems is significant as cognitive flexibility is a necessary component in being able to shift any views that may have developed in maladaptive ways. One's internalized core values and belief systems are important in resiliency in terms of how our perspectives of self, others, and the world impact our responses to stress and behaviors chosen to manage crisis situations when they arise. A family's core values and belief systems create the family's narrative for how stressful situations are to be approached and managed when they arise. These narratives tend to be unspoken, unnoticed, and invisible yet they powerfully guide and shape family interactions and responses to stressful situations often across generations.

Resilience is often discussed in hindsight as a way to understand how an individual, group, or family adapted positively to very difficult life experiences. Resilience is rarely discussed in terms of future (psychosocial) adaptation to stressful life events although it should be a routine part of mental health treatment as prevention against illness. It is not something that someone is born with, or not born with, although certain conditions impact one's ability to respond to stress in more adaptive ways than others. A baby who is born with a temperament that is described as "easy-going" will seek out and accept comfort from their caregivers when they are upset or in distress. The caregivers will feel a degree of confidence in their abilities to provide comfort and a pattern emerges that becomes reinforced and strengthened every time it occurs. Over time, these easy-going babies grow into children who expect that resolution of their distress or upset is not only possible, but is actually probable in their lives given their history of experiencing such interactions. In the absence of any significant negative life events, these children will develop a core belief that the world is a safe place and that not only internal, but external problems as well, will eventually somehow get resolved. This core belief in a healthy resolution of stress provides the foundation when the child expands into their social world outside the family unit. The cognitive belief system that stress and problems are resolved in healthy ways tends to require a certain degree of social skills to achieve this outcome in the circles of school, work, and community life. Core beliefs that problems have

DOI: 10.4324/9781003438229-4

solutions and resiliency can be achieved lead to patterns of functioning in relationships based on these beliefs. In the absence of significant adversity or traumatic life events, resilient children grow into adults who believe that challenging situations are to be expected, problems will be solved, and positive outcomes will be achieved.

Children who live in families and communities that are free from adverse life events have more opportunities to develop this positive feedback loop and often more social supports available to help manage and adapt to stressful experiences. Children who do not have these resources, however, will face more challenges in developing similar cognitive beliefs that the world is a safe place where the environment responds consistently in positive ways. Children who grow up with chronic stress or trauma in their environment will not experience the world as a safe place and this environment plays a major role in challenging even the most resilient children and families. A community's capacity to support resiliency is dependent upon the amount of available resources within that community that can act as protective buffers against stressful situations. An example of this is when children who grow up in large urban settings experience health problems related to over-crowding that impact their ability to be resilient. Children who experience systemic racism and other forms of oppression have considerable risk and adversity to manage on a daily basis and building community capacity for resiliency requires addressing and dismantling these systems of oppression. The ecological theory of systems within systems offers valuable insight into building individual and family resiliency, and building both physical and psychologically healthy communities is one of the most vital aspects in strengthening child and family well-being.

The core of resiliency is a very personal one with meanings that vary across individuals, families, and communities. Resiliency exists in a cultural context that defines what it means to be resilient based on multiple factors that influence and shape the way in which individuals, families, and groups adapt to situations in their lives. Adaptations are deemed healthy when they lead to positive outcomes, such as increased mental health and well-being, and increase one's potential to thrive despite difficult life situations. The notion of resiliency focuses on what it means to adapt to difficult life situations based on the dynamic interplay of many forces that influence and shape our behavioral responses. In order to increase our understanding of what it means to be resilient, we have to deconstruct the outcomes first of the reasons why certain behaviors are chosen over other behaviors in difficult times. If we do not go through this process of deconstructing the outcome, it would be akin to believing that one definition of resiliency fits all people, and all we need to do is figure out a common set of traits shared by seemingly well-adjusted individuals or groups of individuals. The ways that families respond to stressful situations tend to fall into patterns as behaviors chosen in the past signal options for coping with new stressors. This behavioral tendency results from the belief that a coping skill that was effective in the past will be effective again. The notion of resiliency is unique to an individual's lived experiences and situated within the contexts of systemic forces that are in place influencing the ability to be resilient.

The concept of resiliency varies widely and to understand an individual or family's adaptation to stress, without their perspectives and perceptions of the problem, is impossible. The term resilience in certain communities is reflective of that group's ability to employ resistance strategies that empower and create hope through a shared sense of a collective unity to meet life's challenges. The construct of resistance may be in the form of raising the level of collective action engagement in one's community to help build the community's capacity to begin to address inequities in the system. The United States has a history of racial, ethnic, and cultural stratification with policies and practices in place that sustain the marginality of non-dominant groups. Issues of race, gender, and ethnicity impact all areas of military family life, recently reported in terms of military career advancement, as the myth of the military meritocracy was debunked by documented glass ceilings held in place with systemic bias, racism, and oppression. The military has reported recent changes in policies to address the documented glass ceiling in careers, including removing service member photos from promotion packages, however critics have said this will do little to stem the tide of systemic bias that permeates throughout daily military life and that more of an organizational response is required. The core military virtues of collectivism, unity, and positive morale cannot truly exist alongside systemic oppression, privilege, and dominance of one group over others and highlighting this discrepancy could assist in shifting the overall climate to one that is more positive for all members.

The moment that a service member receives notification that he or she is being sent on a deployment starts a series of events for the military family as this moment marks a change that could represent a crisis for the family. In families struggling with food or housing insecurity, the deployment of an adult member of the family can place additional stress and hardship on a family who may have to sacrifice personally in concrete ways to survive. Although a family's income may rise during certain deployments due to hazardous duty pay and tax relief, the loss of the service member and his or her contributions to the safety, stability, and functioning of the family are significant. The perspectives held by the family will influence the choices made in terms of managing any hardships being faced, as well as stress that emerges, and which coping strategies will be employed. While the military service member trains for these types of events throughout their career in the military, the military family has not had such training. There is no training offered to family members for how to manage new roles or demands and support is rarely offered to manage the obstacles and challenges they will encounter. Military spouses are expected to find support among other military spouses in a manner that is largely unorganized and informal in nature. Efforts to make the "force behind the force" (military term for the families) more resilient has recently included ways to make family support more formal with spouses paid for this work that is time-consuming and takes away from other employment opportunities.

As preparations are made for the service member to leave the safety and security of the family unit, wills are drawn up, family care plans created, and many spouses assume Power of Attorney and Health Care Proxy for the service member. During these preparations, anxiety mounts for the family with the reality that the loss could be permanent. The family's belief system is a significant factor in the family's adaptation to the news and this stressor that is suddenly present in daily family life. The family's response is influenced by their perceptions of the situation, with optimism and belief in the future return of the service member crucial parts of family resiliency. In order to assess a family's overall level of resiliency to this stress, and shifting roles in the family system on the horizon, there are concepts and tools for assessing resiliency that could be included during the mobilization stage to more fully prepare the family for the impending separation. There are several areas of family life that impact the system's adaptation to stress, including communication styles and attachment patterns, that can be strengthened through educational efforts to improve the family's resiliency to stress. In addition to these areas, resilient families aim for strength in overall physical health, emotional well-being, formal and informal social networks, and in spiritual parts of life. Resilient families have a shared set of core values that play a key role in resiliency as they bind the family together and create a sense of stability through a shared family identity (Walsh, 2016).

The Military Family Triangle

The hierarchy of the military holds that the needs of the military take precedence over the needs of the service member and the military family. There is a triangle created between the service member, family, and the military who are often in constant conflict with competing demands between the work of the military and the needs of the home and/or family. In some families, the demands of the military are felt as strongly as the presence of an extramarital affair in terms of divided alliances and attention to each group or system. In the Military Family Triangle, the needs of the family and the needs of the military are competing forces in the service member's life that both demand attention. The triangle (service member–family–military) is described by some military service members as similar to what they imagine it would feel like to be in the experience of being in two romantic relationships at the same time. The military life is often compelling and exciting for service members who enjoy their military careers, occupational specialties, and the demanding lifestyle attached to them. The social and emotional bonds in the military form the backbone of the culture and often as strong as the bonds within families. This duality places the service member in the middle of a triangle of loyalty to these two major spheres of life that have equally powerful needs, wants, and demands for time, attention, and emotional attachment.

The role of a military spouse's feelings toward the military is another important area for exploration in resiliency-building as spouses who hold negative feelings toward the military, such as anger for taking their family member away for military work, trainings, or deployments, will permeate the entire family system. A spouse's negative attitude toward the military might also be experienced by younger children in the family as confusing, and in the absence of a developmentally appropriate explanation, this confusion has the potential to increase anxiety for them as a result. Resiliency cannot be understood without discussing risk and protective factors simultaneously as anchor points for understanding a family's ability to adapt to stress. The family's overall response to the notification of an upcoming deployment or geographic move will be influenced by the feelings and perceptions about the deployment and/or the military itself as it impacts the family in transition. Some of the most frequently reported positive impacts to military children of living through the deployment of a parent include positive shifts in their perceptions about themselves. These can include a sense of increased independence, adaptability to new situations and routines, increased resilience, personal growth, and an increased sense of pride. Some of the negative impacts reported include feelings of worry, separation anxiety, difficulty sleeping, nightmares, irritability, and increased aggression (Linsner & Maury, 2021).

Military spouses and family members who hold feelings of anger at the military for a high-risk deployment of the service member will be more likely to experience heightened anxiety that may be difficult to resolve if associated with decreased help-seeking behaviors and a ripple social effect of distancing from other military spouses. Some of the major risk and protective factors that influence resiliency for military spouses are in Figure 2.1. Medical records reviewed from 250,000 spouses of active-duty Army soldiers during deployment included symptoms of depression, anxiety, sleep/adjustment disorders, and acute stress reactions, with longer deployments evidencing higher rates of such symptoms (Mansfield et al., 2010). Some of the of the major risk factors include young age, limited resources, low income levels, and lack of community support due to the constant geographic relocations that erode the sense of stability and forming a community of friends and allies that tend to develop over time.

In addition to feelings around deployments, the notification of an upcoming move to a remote location with limited resources for healthcare, mental health treatment, or disability services may raise feelings of resentment toward the military for a family who may have no control or limited input into the PCS location. In such situations, family members may experience feelings of being trapped in the situation, lacking control over their lives, and/or disempowered by the military. Family notification of a move to a location with different political or social views of the family itself, specifically in terms of education/schooling of children, is likely to raise similar feelings of resentment, disempowerment, and/or anger among family members that will negatively impact the overall climate in the family's home and life environment.

+	-
Sense of Optimism	*Younger Ages (Military Spouse)*
Positive Attitude toward the Military	*Financial Stress*
Deployment Seen as Opportunity	*Making Radical Changes during Deployment*
Time of Personal Development	*Denying the Danger of Service Member*
Taking Responsibility for Personal Preparedness & Self-Determination	*Pile-up of Multiple Stressors*
Channeling Anxiety into Other Activities	*Decreased Community/Social Support*
Developing a Routine	*Mainstream Media and Negative Public Images*
Reaching Out to Others	*Feeling Need to Protect Service Member from Negative Information*
Staying Busy & Not Isolating	

Figure 2.1 Military spouses: protective (+) and risk (-) factors

Military Family Members with Special Needs

In the United States, nearly two million children live in military families and of those children, it is estimated that 20% or more have disabilities (Davis, 2014). On average, military families of children with disabilities use six disability services (ranging from 4–7) per week (Goin-Kochel et al., 2007). Such services include speech, occupational, and physical therapies; social skills groups, medical specialists, and parent training. When children with disabilities receive appropriate services, they experience long-term developmental benefits such as improved cognitive and adaptive functioning and their families experience improved health and well-being. However, military families of children with disabilities often struggle to access needed services, receive timely supports, navigate bureaucracies, and transition into new schools and communities (Aleman-Tovar, 2022). In a study of 189 military families of children with disabilities (Davis et al., 2016), the majority of families reported delays in receiving services (79%); discontinuity of services (69%); delayed child progress due to a lack of services (63%); and difficulty finding medical professionals (59%). In general, 71.3% of military families reported lacking access to needed services for their children with disabilities.

A recent survey of family support providers found that the disabilities reported the most were autism, ADHD (attention-deficit hyperactivity disorder), speech and language disorders, developmental delays, asthma, and mental health problems (Aronson et al., 2016). The Department of Defense oversees the Exceptional Family Member Program (EFMP) to provide support to military families with adult or child dependents who have special medical and/or educational needs, including coordination of support around documenting these needs for the military to consider before finalizing PCS moves. In 2018, more than 132,500 family members enrolled as exceptional family members (U.S. Government Accountability Office, 2018) and it is estimated that approximately two-thirds of dependents in the program are military children. The EFMP is based on the practice of enrollment into the program followed by coordination of the service member's duty assignments following notification of a change in duty station. The service member has two weeks to submit documentation to establish the level of care that is needed for the family members enrolled in the program to appeal the location decision if there is not adequate disability or educational services in the new location. A duty station such as Minot Air Force Base in North

Dakota is an example of one location that tends to be appealed often, due to being located in a remote area with limited access to healthcare resources.

It is common for service members to work six days per week and/or be unable to afford to take or send a family for vacation breaks from a base such as Minot that is geographically isolated. The base at Minot reports high levels of intensity as the base has one of the largest nuclear arsenals of the military. Service members with mental health needs for treatment for themselves or their family members may advocate for a different duty station based on lack of resources available on the base or in the nearest town, which is very small and limited in services. It is up to the base command, however, to decide whether needs can be met or not and since very few service members choose to go to Minot AFB, staffing shortages often dictate these decisions, even for family members with documented histories of mental health needs or disabilities.

The Rehabilitation Act of 1973, the ADA, and the amendments to the ADA have improved conditions for people with disabilities but given that the overwhelming majority of military families report not having needed services for children with disabilities, there are clearly significant changes that need to take place for these children. Families with special needs often require ongoing access to suitable healthcare and specialists and the military is responsible to support the healthcare of family members but especially those with disabilities who have heightened risk factors and vulnerabilities. In addition to healthcare, one of the primary obstacles that families with a child with disabilities encounter is when a family relocates; educational intervention tools, including Individualized Education Plans, and educational accommodation plans (504 Plans), should be continued where the family moves. This does not always happen seamlessly, however, and implementation of those plans can take months to be put into place. This lack of continuity frequently happens with medical care as well and is highly disruptive to a child's development and a major risk factor for all family members with disabilities.

Parent-Focused Families

If you ask a child, adolescent, or adult who has grown up in a military family what they want or need in a therapeutic conversation, the chances are high that they may hesitate or not know how to answer your question. Days, months, and years of habitually focusing on the needs of their military parent, the military family as a functional unit, and the military mission above all else, often leads to difficulty trusting one's instincts for what one may want or need. Military children, even as adults, may have difficulty making independent decisions on their own because they may have limited abilities in this area or may never have developed this skill growing up. Living in a family and environment where no one asks what you want or need on a daily basis has a direct impact on the way that you interact with others and aspects of your personality. Military parents may be reluctant to ask their children what they want in certain situations if they know the answer is likely to be "no" to questions such as "do you want to move again?" If questions such as these come up in family discussions, the outcome often does not change as a result due to the military lifestyle.

In terms of childhood development, military children may grow up believing that feelings are irrelevant in terms of outcomes in family life and life in general. Many military children learn to not trust or give much importance to their feelings as these can be problematic and lead to conflicts in the family. In addition to this, they may develop a lack of trust in their own judgment too. They may respond by going along with people in their lives to avoid conflicts whenever possible and develop a personality style that "goes with the flow" with difficulty expressing or getting their needs met. If this pattern occurs throughout one's life, the military child may grow up to be an adult whose social interactions are positive and free of conflicts although this will tend to be on a superficial behavioral level as the child or grown adult does not experience getting what they want or need in daily life. This child may grow up with feelings that include chronic resentment and feeling devalued on a regular basis as a result of this maladaptive behavioral pattern. These individuals may also be at a loss to understand the etiology (or basis) of such feelings and be confused if psychological symptoms emerge such as anxiety, anger, or constant irritability.

The military family lifestyle and cultural context places the needs of the military and the military service member parent as priorities over the needs of the children and family. In her writing on counseling military families, Hall (2016) draws upon earlier works (Wertsch, 1991) to illustrate the dynamics at work in military family life where the entire family sacrifices, not just the adult caregivers who join, and uses the term "parent-focused families" to describe the system. Military children often experience challenges in the developmental attachment need for safety and trust in their environment that is constantly changing because the family is focused on the needs of the military parent. The current model that has been in operation throughout modern military history is that military family members must suppress their needs to accommodate the needs of the military and the service member by extension that take precedence. This conceptual model holds that military family needs should not interfere with the needs of the military parent's work and career as this model is one where the focus is on the military mission at all times. As a result of this model, military children and family members become indoctrinated into a culture of habitually putting the needs of the military and the military parent ahead of their own needs. Children learn quickly to suppress and detach from their feelings, especially negative ones, as the experience and expression of such needs are often invalidated in the military environment. Growing up in an environment that does not validate one's feelings or experiences leads to a general lack of trust in that environment and the stoic act of appearing to not have any problematic feelings gets validated and reinforced in a positive feedback loop over time. As a result of growing up in an invalidating emotional environment, military children often develop internal frameworks for managing strong emotions through coping behaviors that include suppression and subjugation of their feelings and their needs.

According to Hall (2016) expanding on the work of other theorists, the parenting style that is found in parent-focused families is one of coercive parenting and understood as "limits without freedom." There are rules set for children's behaviors, demands that are often placed on them, and orders that are expected to be followed. There are rewards offered for following the rules and living up to expectations of them. There is a belief in these families that a child does not have a problem that is leading to unhealthy behaviors, but rather that the child is capable of change, and is merely not living up to their potential. Children in these families often learn that it is adaptive for them to detach from their feelings, can become submissive to those in power to make their decisions for them, and not fully develop independent life skills. As there is little tolerance for questioning the authority of one's parents, there may be frequent violations of children's privacy due to the fact that the parents believe they have a need to know everything that is going on at all times. Children are often discouraged from individuation from the family unit which often works during early childhood and through the elementary school years. When children become teenagers, and need to individuate as part of the developmental stage of adolescence, family conflicts arise when they leave base for civilian high schools, interact with civilian teenagers, and experience a different way of relating to adults and with the world.

Permissive parenting is the opposite style and can be understood as "freedom without limits" and operates in child-focused families where children are treated as princes and princesses and the parents are there to serve them at all times, meet all of their needs, wants, and desires and sacrifice their own. Children in these families have a deep sense of entitlement as they never have to earn their rewards, they have limited social skills, overly depend on others, and lack self-discipline. Parents in these families eventually come to resent how much they are doing for their children and these families experience power struggles and family conflicts when there are rules and expectations for social behaviors placed on the children. Respectful leadership parenting is a healthy medium between the other two extreme forms of parenting and understood as "freedom within limits." This style of parenting creates a feeling of safety for children with boundaries designed to protect them and not to suffocate their individual growth within the family system. The parents are seen as the leaders in the family, leading with mutual respect in all of the family's interactions with one another, and with the outside world. The parents build on the strengths and highlight the positives of the children and the family as both an effective and functional system. The family promotes responsibility and instills confidence based on the positive traits of all of the individuals and the family as a whole. Through a sense of fairness and personal responsibility to the group, these parents create a sense of mutual interdependence and the children tend to grow up to be respectful of the needs of others while taking care of their own individual needs at the same time.

Childhood Schemas and Coping Styles

Schema therapy is based on the notion that there are schemas, or cognitive templates, developed during childhood and adolescence that are based on a child's interactions with caregivers (Young et al., 2003). Schemas operate on an unconscious level out of our awareness and help to form our coping styles in life as well as our sense of self and our expectations about the world and our relationships. This therapy model targets the developmental origins of behaviors that were adaptive coping responses in childhood and adolescence that become maladaptive and problematic patterns of psychosocial functioning later in life. In adulthood, patterns of interacting with the world are embedded into one's personality and the aspects that are problematic will lead to repetitive, chronic, and long-term conditions and dissatisfaction in terms of achieving happiness. The schema therapy model entails three areas of psychological functioning: schemas are the core themes; coping styles are the behavioral responses to those schemas; and modes describe the interaction of maladaptive schemas and coping styles (Young et al., 2003). According to the schema therapy model, based on cognitive behavioral therapy models, there are 18 maladaptive schemas and these can be explored through psychotherapeutic means. Early maladaptive schemas that were based on childhood perceptions of self, others, and the environment lead to coping behaviors in response to these interactions that can continue throughout one's life and allow the distress to remain active and present (Martin & Young, 2010).

Maladaptive schemas include adverse childhood experiences that result in negative cognitions or beliefs about self, others, and the world and the therapy model targets these negative perceptions (Martin & Young, 2010). Schema therapy often focuses on one or more of the following areas: abandonment by caregivers resulting in instability in the home environment; mistrust from child abuse; emotional deprivation leading to the belief that all people are selfish; feeling defective from shaming interactions; social isolation and feelings of alienation or being different from others; being overly dependent on others resulting in incompetency; believing one is vulnerable to harm or illness and unsafe in the world as a result; being enmeshed with caregivers leading to an undeveloped sense of self and lacking a sense of one's identity as independent from caregivers; feeling as if one is a failure and disappointment to caregivers; believing one is entitled to special treatment from a sense of grandiosity; believing one lacks self-control or self-discipline; believing one has to subjugate or suppress one's needs resulting in the individual not knowing what they need or want and feeling angry on a daily basis but unaware of the reason; believing one must self-sacrifice and take care of other people's needs before their own needs; seeking approval or recognition from others on a continual basis; pervasive feelings of negativity or pessimism that people will let people down; believing that one must inhibit or restrict one's emotions because they are dangerous or unpredictable; believing that one must live up to unrelenting standards from having highly critical caregivers; and belief that one deserves punishments for behaviors that don't live up to expectations of caregivers (Martin & Young, 2010).

As childhood behavioral patterns based on maladaptive schemas become entrenched in behaviors that no longer meet the needs and demands of the environment where they emerged, therapy focuses on challenging these beliefs about one's self at the core. Schema therapy was developed as an offshoot of cognitive behavioral therapy as the goals of both include shifting negative perceptions or cognitive distortions to more positive ones that then influence the behaviors one chooses based on them. Adulthood is filled with interactions based on early childhood schemas, and when these are from negative situations in one's home environment, those interactions are likely to cause distress or psychological symptoms to emerge as a result. Behavioral adaptations that were concretized and set into one's character and personality from adversity in childhood or adolescence often lead to functional impairments later in life when the demands for autonomy and competency take precedence.

When negative childhood schemas are perpetuated into adulthood, they are often no longer necessary or accurate in relation to the situation and their dysfunctional nature becomes apparent (Martin & Young, 2010). Adult schemas are triggered by life events that the person perceives as being similar to childhood events and the person experiences strong negative emotions such as grief, shame, fear, or rage. The more severe schemas are activated more often by a number of situations and lead to more intense and longer-lasting negative affective states. Since schemas influence how individuals think, feel, behave, and interact socially, if they are never brought into conscious awareness and challenged on an intellectual level, they will remain intact, shaping how that person understands their experiences and their world. Schemas are familiar and comfortable cognitive perceptions that are usually rigid and not flexible because of a long history of "self-fulfilling prophecies" that reinforce them over and over again. Individuals are drawn to people and situations that trigger their schemas in a process known as "schema chemistry" where the schema responsible for one's behaviors is believed to be true and feels comfortable even when it is the cause of much pain and suffering.

"Schema perpetuation" describes the psychodynamic process that an individual goes through internally and behaviorally that maintains the schema and includes thoughts, feelings, actions, and interactions with others. Adults who repeatedly find themselves in situations that are painful, unfulfilling, or not meeting their stated goals in life are often attempting to succeed in achieving the developmental tasks of being an adult with the beliefs and behaviors of a child. The adult who wants to break this cycle of destructive patterns that emerge and continuously prevent them from achieving their goals in life needs to first bring maladaptive schemas into conscious awareness to be able to then shift the cognitive beliefs that accompany them. Cognitive behavioral therapy is present-focused and it is generally considered impossible to shift behaviors and cognitive beliefs without addressing the interactional relationship template where they developed.

Children who grow up in military families often develop childhood schemas or frameworks that are represented in parent-focused families where the military demands took priority over child wishes or needs. The schema that has been referred to as the "subjugation schema" is one where childhood needs are subjugated to parental needs and in the case of military children, childhood needs are regularly subjugated to the needs of the military as family life is dictated by the military. Military children grow up not knowing what they want or need simply because they never developed the ability to identify these because it was never part of their family life. Military children are rarely asked if they want to move to a new duty station, or if they want their military parent to be sent on a high-risk deployment and live without that parent for an extended period. Adults who do not know what they want or need on a daily basis have great difficulty achieving the sense of independence that is necessary for fulfilling the demands of adulthood. Oftentimes, military children remain more comfortable being part of a larger unit, team, or family of origin simply because they have never considered what they want as separate individuals with their own needs and independent goals.

The subjugation schema includes the belief that one's emotions, needs, preferences, and opinions are not important, and if emotions are not suppressed, they will cause rejection or punishment. One's feelings and desires are not suppressed because of values or standards, but because of fear that something bad will happen if they are not suppressed. Adults with this schema usually allow others to dominate them and often enter into relationships with controlling partners where they feel weak and powerless and may even become rebellious to counteract these vulnerable feelings and negative beliefs. Schema therapy with the subjugation model (based on the treatment model of Martin and Young, 2010) targets the cognitive realm by challenging the perceived (exaggerated) negative consequences of expressing one's own needs without thinking of the family as a unit and the needs of the parents as primary. One piece of therapy for a child who grows up in a parent-focused family would be for the child to be able to express the chronic anger and irritability that has been experienced and assert their feelings often through the use of imagery. In terms of behavioral changes, the child who grows up in a parent-focused family (including the military child and as a grown adult) would have goals that include selecting non-controlling partners (who tolerate and even encourage them to assert their needs) and learning to trust their instincts to be able to effectively act on them. In the therapy relationship, the therapist would be careful not to be controlling and would encourage them to make their own decisions and choices regularly; the therapist would point out times that they did not express what they wanted or needed in situations and identify anger as a response to these patterns of deference based on the early maladaptive schema of subjugation of needs.

The Military Lifestyle and Child Development

In the two decades spanning the post-9/11 wars, more than two million American (U.S.) children lived through a parent's deployment and more than 800,000 lived through two or more deployments. Longer deployments and shorter dwell times were risk factors for overall distress and mental health problems with children who had parents deployed from National Guard/Reserve units (approximately 750,000 children) considered at increased risk due to being isolated from other military children without a normalizing structure for the military lifestyle. Approximately 75% of children of U.S. service members are under the age of 11 years and in a critical stage of childhood development to be exposed to heightened, sometimes damaging, levels of stress in their homes and families. Twice as many children in military families report anxiety as compared with civilian children and more than one-third have demonstrated elevated emotional or behavioral problems. These children may learn how to cope with the stress while it is happening, but if left untreated, these reactions and behaviors can worsen into significant mental health diagnoses and disorders lasting long into adulthood.

The Military Child Education Coalition's Student-2-Student program trains civilian and military-connected high school and middle-school students to establish and sustain peer-based programs in their schools to support military children as they regularly transition to and from new schools. The program aims to create support networks for youths and provide military children with immediate peer credibility, positive peer relationships, and valuable information about the school and the community. The program developed in light of the fact that every school district in the United States has military-connected children. In civilian communities, there can be children of active-duty service members, or members of the Army or Air Force National Guard units, or members of reserve units across every branch of service. There are approximately two million military children as well as almost double that number when you include youths with veterans as parents. Military family connectedness and participation in this prevention program were significantly associated with higher positive youth development and lower depressive symptoms. Research suggests that being in a military family has the potential to be a context for thriving due to the many strengths and opportunities to practice, reinforce, and hone the necessary skills of adaptation associated with the military lifestyle. For example, every geographic relocation that a military child makes is an opportunity for growth depending on how that child and family perceive, approach, and manage the situation.

Parents and caregivers who encourage children to develop friendships, however short-lived and role model doing so themselves, create family habits that are positive responses to situations that are less than favorable or stressful in some way. Developing friendships throughout childhood are crucial social skills necessary for bonding and forming attachments outside of the family which youth need to accomplish as one of the achievements of healthy development. Children and adolescents who do not fully develop these skills for forming strong bonds outside of the family are likely to run into challenges when they need to separate from their family-of-origin in early adulthood and begin independent lives and/or new families of their own. In addition to forming these friendships during a military child's life, caregivers, teachers, coaches, and therapists all need to encourage and role-model conflict resolution for military children who often don't develop these critical social skills as well.

Why is conflict resolution a necessary skill to learn in a child's development? Children who don't learn how to negotiate difficult situations that are filled with conflict never learn how to maintain attachment bonds with their peers that are crucial aspects of supporting resiliency through building one's social community. In addition to providing an emotional buffer in times of stress, resolving conflicts within one's social networks is a skill that is necessary for strengthening and maintaining a community that is effective in meeting the needs of all its members. Communities of one's peers, regardless of the age or stage of development, are vital for sustaining the ability to overcome challenges and manage stress when difficult situations arise. The ability to resolve conflicts with peers also helps children learn how to prevent disruptions in attachment bonds that serve as mediating and restorative roles when overwhelming emotional states arise. Attachment bonds with peers can also serve to provide a safe haven for military families struggling with familial attachment disruptions during a wartime deployment and help to prevent the transmission of inter-generational traumatic stress that may result in military families.

In terms of resiliency, individual characteristics combine with one's social contexts, relationships, perceptions about adversity, and the capacity to manage difficult situations. Strengths found in resilient youth from military families are those that are able to meet the demands of the military lifestyle and family adversity that can result from the pile-up of demands including geographic moves and deployment separations. Adolescents from military families would benefit from programs designed to enhance the strengths of teens in this stage of development. The pieces of resiliency that are necessary in meeting chronic demands include the following attributes of psychosocial functioning: cognitive and emotional flexibility; ability to regulate one's emotions internally; having an internal locus of control and sense of agency with behavioral self-regulation; a sense of humor; hopefulness and optimism; good health; and being born with a baseline and overall easy-going temperament to respond to stressful situations in life. Family relationships that are based on secure attachments help children make meaning out of adversity as they feel connected and a sense of belonging that is protective in nature. Youth who are connected in their family by a set of clear and spoken values are able to understand adversity and feel empowered to meet such demands when they arise in light of these shared values.

Strengths found in active-duty military families include feeling a sense of purpose, identity, and belonging as being part of the military community that is often not present in the civilian communities of the National Guard and Reserves. Many important resources needed by the family are provided by the military to active-duty military families as well as the presence of a built-in social support system and unwaveringly strong structure/foundation provided to families by military life. Social supports provided on military bases to active-duty families typically include recreational facilities, pools, movie theaters, bowling alleys, social events, religious services, and regularly scheduled activities for children and families. Some of the significant guiding precepts associated with military life and the ethos of military culture that impact family resiliency include the commitment to duty to the military mission and are often described as doing what is necessary and/or right regardless of personal costs. This commitment to military service and duty that takes priority over family life often leads service members, spouses, and their children to develop an increased tolerance for frustration, disappointment, and an overall acceptance of what cannot be changed in situations. The daily practice of assessing situations to determine what can be changed or altered, and accepting what is not negotiable in any given situation, allows for a cognitive appraisal of the situation to take shape quickly. Military families tend to possess highly developed abilities for assessing situational awareness which influences the meaning that one then attributes to the (personal or familial) manageability of the situation. An example of this can be seen when a service member receives PCS orders to a new location, and the family must problem-solve collaboratively about what they have control over (whether they live on the military base or in the civilian community) as well as what they do not have control over (where the service member will be working). Situations such as this occur routinely in military family life and influence a family's overall ability to tolerate frustration and develop skills for adaptive coping based on heightened abilities for cognitively constructing realistic appraisals based on information presented to them.

In terms of risk factors, military families adapt to change on a regular basis and do so without the presence of older relatives, friends, or neighbors living on military bases to offer the guidance, wisdom, and diverse perspectives that come from living among an inter-generational community. Older community members who may be retired are often able to offer a balanced perspective on life in general and sometimes provide free child-care to a young family in need. Grand-parenting is generally seen as a positive influence on children as grandparents tend not to have the same expectations that parents have which can allow children to experience a caregiving experience that is very different than the one they have with their parents. Children who have strong attachments to caregivers who have less expectations and demands of them are able to see themselves through these caregivers' eyes, which can be a very positive experience for them. Military families endure constant change, challenges, and new situations in their lives and would benefit greatly from having the availability of an extended network of relatives to support them.

Positive Youth Development

Despite the challenges of the lifestyle and the lack of extended support networks, military children often thrive and demonstrate adaptive resilience in the midst of multiple layers of stressful situations. In previous decades, theories around adolescent development tended to focus on a deficit model for the teenage years that held that impulses were negative forces that needed to be controlled. Theories were often linear in nature much like that of dominoes where problems in one stage caused a ripple effect in the ones that followed next in line. The "lead domino" theory sets in motion a series of events that propel the rest of one's life in one direction or another without factoring in the multiple layers of context and relationships that intervene along the way. In development across the life cycle, Eric Erickson's model states that there are eight key developmental milestones throughout the course of one's life from birth through death with task completion necessary for each stage. In this model, individuals who do not complete the developmental tasks of any given stage will be more likely to run into problematic situations in the next stage as a result. These stages proceed from birth to death including childhood (early, middle, and adolescence) and adulthood (young adult, middle-aged adult, and older adult). The specific tasks and ages as described by Erikson's model (listed below) include the ones that are specific to military service members of late adolescence and young adulthood of forming an identity and establishing strong affiliative and social bonds in relationships. Veterans who transition out of military service after a full career in the military will be in the stage of middle adulthood when struggles with stagnation can arise if an individual does not have a sense of purpose or feel productive and generative in one's life.

1 Early infancy: trust vs. mistrust (1–1 ½ years)
2 Toddler: autonomy vs. shame and doubt (1 ½ –3 years)
3 Early childhood: initiative vs. guilt (3–6 years)
4 Middle childhood: industry vs. inferiority (6–12 years)
5 Adolescence: identity vs. identity confusion (12–18 years)
6 Early adulthood: intimacy vs. isolation (19–40 years)
7 Middle adulthood: generativity vs. stagnation (40–65 years)
8 Older adulthood: integrity vs. despair (65 years and older)

Positive Youth Development (PYD) is a term that emerged in recent decades as a conceptual approach that factored in biology, developmental science, and relational theories and focused on areas of strengths in childhood and adolescence (Bowers et al., 2014). Theories and research of PYD challenged the notion that adolescence was a tumultuous phase filled with emotional storms that needed to be contained at all costs as if they were dangerous, unpredictable, and risky. The concept of PYD offered ways of understanding adolescence as a positive opportunity for growth that could buffer stress and prevent depressive symptoms. In terms of child development, resilience involves the ability to engage in adaptive behaviors that allow a child to achieve developmental milestones despite facing significant stressful situations or traumatic life events. The characteristics of a youth's personality that influence developmental outcomes include the areas of competence, confidence, connection, character, and caring (Bowers et al., 2014). The main organizing theory of PYD is that all adolescents have strengths known as developmental assets and all of their contexts have resources that can contribute to resilience and healthy development. The assets found in families, schools, faith institutions, youth-serving organizations, and the communities where they engage in interactive social relations are crucial aspects of positive development. When the strengths of youth combine with developmental assets found in their social relationships, adaptive responses to stress occur and resiliency flourishes.

Key areas of ecological influence for positive youth development include individual people such as mentors, family members, teachers, physical environments, and institutional resources such as parks, schools, and community-based programs. PYD is an adaptive developmental process that involves bi-directional relations between the attributes of youth and their environments of family, school, and communities (Geldhof, Bowers, & Lerner, 2013). The five aspects referred to as the "5 Cs of PYD" illustrated in Figure 2.2 include connection, competence, confidence, character, and caring and are all critical components of healthy youth development (Lerner et al., 2018). According to this model, positive development occurs when there is an alignment between the strengths of the individual (including intentional self-regulation skills, hopefulness for the future, and active engagement in school) and their positive environmental contexts that serve as developmental assets (including warmth and involvement from parents or sustained relationships with caring and competent mentors or youth program workers). This strengths-based approach to youth development is a key feature to understanding adolescent resiliency and thriving in the midst of adversity. Although adolescents spend increasingly more time with their peers than with their parents, most adolescents still value their relationships with their parents and significant adult mentors in their lives enormously. For the most part, adolescents have core values that are consistent with those of their parents including the importance of education in one's life as well as views on social justice and spirituality. Most adolescents also tend to select friends who share similar core values to those of their families.

Positive and sustained adult–youth relationships are one of the most significant hallmarks of positive youth development, combined with programs that build life skills, and the availability of opportunities for youth to participate in leadership positions in family, school, and community activities. Three characteristics significantly influence youth development in positive ways: intentional self-regulation; hope for the future; and engagement in school across behavioral, emotional, and

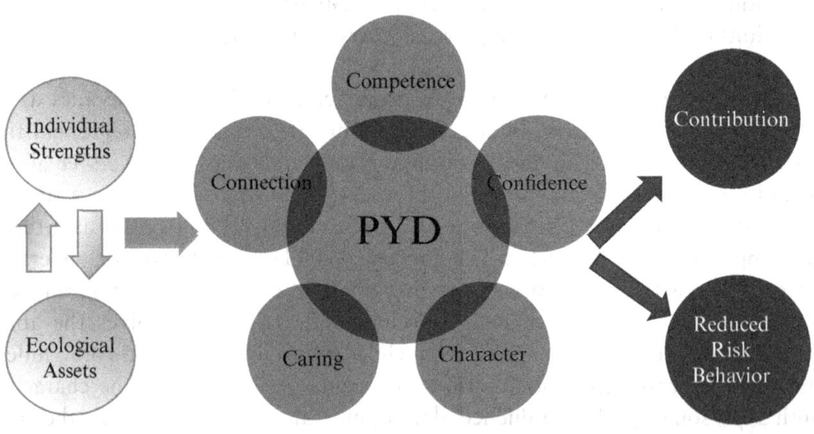

Figure 2.2 The 5 Cs of Positive Youth Development (PYD) Model (Lerner et al., 2018)

cognitive domains. An important outcome of positive development is being active and engaged in civic areas of participation including civic duty, civic skills, and in one's neighborhood and social connections. Other significant outcomes of positive youth development include: reduced depression, problematic risk behaviors, delinquency, and substance use; higher academic outcomes; and increased engagement and contribution across the many communities that individuals interact with on a regular basis.

Positive Youth Development has been operationalized into programs that promote healthy adolescent development through focusing on specific aspects of this stage that is one of plasticity and open to change. In terms of specific aspects of personality development that are crucial to include for programs designed to enhance positive youth development, specific areas need to be considered. PYD programs target the following aspects of development: they promote bonding and build competence across social, emotional, cognitive, behavioral, and moral areas; they foster resilience, self-determination, spirituality, self-efficacy, a clear and positive identity, and a hopeful belief in the future. PYD programs recognize positive behaviors and create opportunities for social involvement that is positive and situated within cultural norms. Bonding refers to the emotional attachment and commitment a child makes to their family, peers, school, community, culture. Resilience is a child's capacity for adapting to change and stressful events in healthy and flexible ways. Competency refers to developing skills that can integrate feelings, thinking, and behaviors that help children achieve goals. Behavioral competency includes using behaviors in positive ways that are effective in helping an individual achieve their stated goals. Specific areas of behavioral competency include non-verbal communication (facial expressions, tone of voice, how one is dressed, appearance, gestures, eye contact); verbal communication (clear and direct requests and expressions of emotions to others; effective responses to actual and perceived criticism); and taking action (walking away from negative situations; participating in positive activities; and helping others when needed). Moral competency is the ability to respond to ethical, affective, and social-justice situations in appropriate ways with empathy, a respect for rules, and knowing the clear distinction between right and wrong (Catalano et al., 2004).

Given the military culture's strict guidelines for behavior that reflect one's values, the tenets of Positive Youth Development fit perfectly well into the military lifestyle and programs for children, youth, and adolescents. As military service members are indoctrinated into service with a clear set of honor codes, values, and beliefs about overcoming adversity, military families often share similar values and belief systems. As a result of growing up in a military family, military youth often perceive adversity in similar ways to their parents and respond to difficult life situations based on their family's values and belief system. Military youth who grow up in families that openly discuss the values of character, integrity, and honor on a regular basis and live according to these values in times of stress learn to perceive difficulty through this lens. Military families that discuss the meaning of the value of honor, for example, and what it means to be an honorable person, raise children who grow up seeing this value put into actionable behavior on a consistent and regular basis. Military children hear, learn, and internalize beliefs about values on a daily basis, by word and by example, in their families and the wider military community in every social interaction including traditions, events, and ceremonies that incorporate such values into everyday life. In this way, military children may easily perceive being given the responsibility for a task or taking care of another family member as an honorable thing to do rather than a burden that is put upon them.

Families Responding to Notification Orders (Case Study)

A military family stationed in California received notification orders of a move to a different state they had never been to before so the military spouse reached out to her network of military spouses on the new base's social media page to find out more about housing options and anything else that might be helpful. She heard from a spouse who had lived on that base while housing was similar to most bases, the school environment was very different than the one their two children were attending at the time. The spouse was informed that she should meet with school staff to go over the rules since there were options for parents to choose in terms of disciplinary actions if behavior ever warranted intervention. This was concerning to the parents because their younger child had recently been diagnosed with Attention Deficit Hyperactivity Disorder (ADHD) after impulsively throwing a shoe in class that nearly missed the teacher. The spouse had heard that it was possible that their children would not get the services they needed in the classroom because the school "did not believe in ADHD" and believed that it represented a lack of discipline at home and in school. Reports were that the school offered parents the option of "opting out" of their practice of paddling children who were disruptive behaviorally.

The parents began looking for housing outside the base in the civilian community where they felt they would have more control over school choices but found that housing prices were too high for the family given the service member's income level. The family made phone calls to private schools in the community so that they could drive the children to schools off base, and were shocked to find that they were higher than the rental prices for housing on base. The service member made the decision to speak with his commanding officer to seek a different location but was unable to change as his training requirements demanded that he go to that location as there were no other locations that could provide the training he needed. The parents experienced different reactions to the information and the service member took the view that it was out of their control so they "would just make the best of it" and see what happened. The spouse, however, was angry and frustrated with the military for not having schools with a more uniform system of schooling and being forced to move to a state with social and political views that were very different than those of their family. She was anxious and worried that her child would be teased or bullied in the new location and felt a complete lack of control over her parenting choices concerning the health, mental health, and education of their children. She became frustrated with her spouse for his response to "make the best of it" and they began to argue on a daily basis with no results to their arguments. These different views regarding the stressful situation led the parents and entire family to have a difficult time adapting to the transition so they began counseling that was encouraged by the service member's command. The parents attended short-term therapy that was focused on finding solutions to problems (solution-focused brief therapy) which turned out to be a perfect fit for them because it focused on their strengths as a couple and as a family. They were able to figure out solutions based on their unique coping skills that they had used in previous stressful situations and became more effective in the ways in which they were communicating with each other. They were able to collaboratively problem solve and came to the decision that the spouse would stop working and home-school the children for the duration of the PCS move.

3 Assessing Family Capacity to Manage Stress

Strengthening Resiliency: Emotions and Tasks

Military families offer valuable insights into resiliency through the constant adaptations they are forced to endure such as routine transitions among roles and role responsibilities due to military work-related demands. Different coping strategies have been found to contribute to different outcomes and different levels of overall well-being and resiliency as a result of behavioral choices made when faced with a stressful situation. One study conducted with military spouses previously mentioned found that those who employed task-oriented coping were able to divert their attention away from difficult or painful emotions by staying focused on achieving their goals as a behavioral adaptation to stress (Wang et al., 2018). This study reported that emotion-oriented coping is a strategy that is focused on changing negative or painful feelings associated with a problematic situation in an effort to reduce the associated stress. The alternative, task-oriented coping, is a strategy in which the individual takes actions in an effort to alter the problematic situation that is causing the stress. The shift from being problem-focused to being task-focused is similar to the guiding principles found in the strengths-based perspective of solution-focused brief therapy (SFBT). Military spouses who used emotion-focused coping strategies were reported to have more difficulty resolving their negative feelings, and experienced higher degrees of depression, than those who created and employed task-oriented behavioral goals during stressful situations (Wang et al., 2018).

The military employs several strengths-based training programs to build resiliency for service members and military families and often turns to positive psychology (Seligman, 2002) to develop these trainings. Marines have utilized the Combat Operational Stress Continuum Model (COSC) in understanding the areas of health, wellness, and resiliency. In this model, there are color-coded zones across the functional areas of life: Green (Ready to Go) is the equivalent of having no stress in one's life; Yellow (Reacting) means that there is mild stress; Orange (Injured) signals that the individual has been damaged by stress and is at risk for failure to perform the roles or duties expected of them; Red (experiencing severe illness) designates that there is a diagnosed mental health disorder including: posttraumatic stress disorder, various forms of depression or anxiety, and/or substance use disorders.

The other branches of service have also developed resiliency trainings over time such as Master Resilience Training (MRT) courses for service members to teach other service members resiliency skills. Battleground Mindset was an Army program used to assist service members during the reintegration period following a stressful deployment to a combat zone with a focus on family resiliency that was direct and to the point. Military One Source, the official Department of Defense resource for military family members, openly states on their website that "Resilient families are flexible, connected and great at using their resources to solve problems." It advises families that ways to build resiliency are to "Listen and show affection, get connected, get comfortable with change, and stay

DOI: 10.4324/9781003438229-5

positive." All of these reflect the military culture of strength in the face of adversity and are perfectly in sync with the solution-focused approach for adaptation to stressful life events. Positive psychology holds that happiness and emotional satisfaction are achieved by identifying, nurturing, and practicing one's unique strengths on a daily basis including optimism, kindness, generosity, and humor (Seligman, 2002). The guiding philosophy of positive psychology is that the practice of continually focusing on our strengths and not our weaknesses causes the weaknesses to wither from lack of attention. The metaphor of strengthening muscles by using them regularly is useful in the internal resiliency metaphor as healthy, adaptive responses to stress can be developed by continued use of them. The old adage for physical health in terms of healthy muscles that states "use it or lose it" can be applied to resiliency in terms of adapting to stress with adaptations that have worked well in the past. The less one uses and focuses on one's strengths, the less likely they will do so in future situations. The more often an individual practices healthy responses to stress, the more they believe that they are competent to manage obstacles. The practice of responding to stress from a perception of strength rather than weakness repeatedly builds confidence to manage stressful situations when they arise that in turn alters the outcome of situations in healthy ways.

The military tradition to hold a ceremony before leaving for a deployment is one of the rituals that is universal for all military service members and often with their families as witness to the ceremonial farewell. While this experience is designed to be affirming and comforting, as aspects of coming together in a large community can be solidifying and less isolating, it can also be challenging for families as they say goodbye publicly in front of other people. Military service members who participate in such ceremonies are seen in formation by their family members as part of the cohesive military group that also strengthens the group's identity as warriors going into battle. At the same time as the warrior identity is being strengthened as a cohesive and functioning unit, service members are ceremoniously moved away from the identity as a family member in order to do so. Military families often experience this shift during such ceremonies and become acutely aware of the transition of the service member out of the family unit and into the military organization. As military families prepare to say goodbye, they quickly realize they are saying goodbye to the family member they know, who is now standing in front of them as a warrior, shoulder to shoulder with other warriors, and the experience changes everyone. The influence of ceremonial traditions in the military such as these is to provide a sense of stability and minimize emotional uncertainty, chaos, or confusion. In addition to maintaining stability for the service members transitioning to the deployment, the experience aims to provide stability for family members as being part of a collective community of families experiencing the same event. The experience of being in a community experiencing the same or similar feelings offers families relief that it is shared with other family members. Difficult emotions that are experienced in isolation can often feel less normative than those experienced in a community or public group situation. As in all military traditions, from the deployment send-off to all the change notifications along the way, there are emotions associated that hold the potential to be overwhelming to individuals and the family system. Military families must negotiate stressful and changing situations on a regular basis and doing so often requires managing emotions so they do not overwhelm the family's ability to function at optimal levels.

The military is mission-driven and relies on an organizational structure that supports achieving those missions as its primary objective. The overall emotions associated with being mission-driven need to support this objective in order to be successful for service members and the family members who live with them on a daily basis. The relationships that make up one's immediate family network of daily interactions and a functioning system are impacted in direct ways by the demands of the military and its constantly changing lifestyle. These immediate family relationships form the attachment network that needs to sustain a measure of balance in order to continue to function at the highest level. The nature of family functioning is one that is made of competing demands among family members and the process of assessing which demands take priority at any given time are always negotiated. Families that function at optimal levels have often done so through daily repetitions of responses to one another that work best for the entire system and no one individual member. There are three key areas that operate in families that can be assessed and strengthened to increase functional capacity and resiliency to stress: the family's belief systems and values; the family's organizational patterns; and the family's communication processes (Walsh, 2016).

Family Resiliency: Beliefs and Core Values

Resilient families make meaning out of adversity, learn from it, and grow as a result; they view crisis situations as manageable, understandable to all family members, and a challenge that is shared together with a positive outlook no matter how large the crisis might be. Resilient families have a shared confidence about overcoming challenges, a strong sense of family cohesiveness, a shared belief that life is meaningful, manageable, and explicable to all members, and an overall sense of optimism about the present situation as well as future situations (Walsh, 2016). The literature on resiliency in families translates well to military family life due to the unique culture of the military in multiple ways including: the belief in the family as a unit that works together as a team and not as independent individuals; the belief that all obstacles can be overcome with the strengths of the team coming together; the belief that situations can be explained to all members of the hierarchy in different yet shared ways; the military's belief that the team is working toward a better outcome and a brighter future (seen in career progressions and building teams based on collective and individual strengths). Families need a narrative to explain their story to themselves and to others that is based in the belief that they have overcome obstacles in the past, mastered them together, and will take these skills with them into the future.

Some of the significant worldviews and adaptations that can strengthen family resilience prior to the moment of a crisis, such as a deployment looming on the horizon, include a shared sense of family cohesiveness based on the family's values and confidence that they can manage the situation. On a daily basis, some protective factors include the family having positive outlooks on life in general and trust in their support systems of extended family, friends, neighbors, and people in their various communities such as work and school. Families that are resilient tend to have a clear family identity that is based on their history, values, strengths, and shared belief systems. Adaptations that families make during stressful situations that weaken the system's strength and overall resiliency include breakdowns in the functioning of the system that challenges the family's beliefs about themselves and lead to negative interactions that divide the family rather than unite its members. The most useful time to strengthen a family's beliefs about their capacity to manage stress is before a crisis occurs and before complications arise that make resiliency more difficult. Families that are prepared to manage emergencies are more resilient in managing the external stress as well as the internal stress that can arise between family members during the response to the crisis.

Resilient families often have beliefs that are culturally syntonic with military life including the focus on health and strength and never wanting to be the "weak link" in one's self-concept. The military culture views challenges as opportunities for growth; has a sense of optimism, perseverance, bravery, and courage in the face of distress; the culture is based on an overall sense of discipline of behavior and emotions, hard work to overcome challenges, and the importance of modulating and/or controlling one's reactions and responses that accompanies the value of stoicism. Positive psychology that includes optimism is a good fit for military family resiliency as the ability to modulate stress through affect regulation skills provides competency and a sense of mastery that are important areas of resiliency. The ability to regulate one's emotions affords a sense of control during a crisis and is an important area in the military's cultural code for manners and behaviors that are key features in resilient responses to stressful situations.

Family Resiliency: Organizational Patterns

The second area of family resiliency covers organizational patterns as resilient families have patterns that are made up of flexibility and cohesiveness of the family as a unit and are able to mobilize social and economic resources when they are needed (Walsh, 2016). They are able to adapt to stress and reorganize to regain stability quickly with respect among family members and a sense of strong leadership in the system. Resilient families have communication that is clear and consistent and clarifies ambiguous information; there is open emotional expression of both painful and positive feelings; there is active collaborative problem-solving and a proactive stance that focuses on goal attainment in the future with concrete steps taken that learn from mistakes and build on successes. This area is culturally syntonic with the military culture in the following ways: the necessary flexibility of roles and responsibilities when needed as evidenced in the constantly changing military lifestyle and in meeting the demands that deployments place on family life; the military family operates as a cohesive unit reflecting the military culture and ethos; and social and economic resources are necessary in times of stress for support as the military relies on developing strength in the family's informal and formal support networks to achieve more than they could as isolated nuclear families without such networks.

Family Resiliency: Communication

Resilient families have open clarity in their communications with one another, open and honest emotional expression, and collaborative problem solving as a team (Walsh, 2016). Communication is the third and final area of family resiliency that resonates well with military families who have the capacity to strengthen this area of resiliency prior to a crisis due to this cultural fit. The collectivist nature of the military culture supports open and direct communication, collaborative problem-solving to work together to tackle problems, and individuals not making decisions on their own in a vacuum when such decisions impact multiple people in their family. Clarity is one of the main strengths that can be found or developed in military families in that the military encourages being direct and open in all areas of one's life from career issues to personal problems. Families who do not feel comfortable with people outside the family unit being involved in matters of family life often have difficulty with this aspect of military life where privacy is often impossible, especially for families living on active-duty bases.

Naming Core Values in Times of Stress

The process of naming core values with families often provides a stabilizing force in times of stress or in the midst of a family crisis. Core values often illuminate the way forward for families who may be stuck in emotional responses to one another or uncertain of tasks that are needed to achieve their overall unified goals. The process of identifying core values is often easier to achieve when done in times of relative calm to be able to identify these to return to in crisis situations. Resiliency is best achieved when adaptations and behavioral choices are made that are in alignment with core values for individual family members and the family as a system. The absence of being able to identify one's core values makes it difficult to know what choices to make in times of challenging or stressful situations and often leads to choices that are not resilient as a result.

The practice of naming core family values assists in unifying a family and adding a buffer against stress in times of chaos or confusion. In the realm of positive psychology theory, individuals and families who live according to their core values have demonstrated increased resiliency against stress, anxiety, and symptoms of depression. An assessment tool that identifies and measures living by one's values in the midst of adversity was developed for the four domains of work/education, leisure time activities, relationships, and personal growth/health (Lundgren et al., 2012). The tool places these domains into a visual dartboard to identify and track progress toward achieving a life that is consistent with one's personal values. This exercise can help individuals identify the obstacles that are getting in the way of living a life that is consistent with their value system through narrative descriptions that have prevented their family from being resilient in times of stress in the past.

Measuring Resiliency: The Military Genogram

Three very useful tools in establishing a family's level of resiliency are the military genogram (Weiss et al. 2010), the Walsh Family Resilience Questionnaire (Walsh, 2016), and the creation of a family timeline. These assessment tools include resilience-based themes about family relationships, cultural influences, and intergenerational narratives that are a perfect fit for the military family. A healthcare provider and/or family member are able to identify the areas of strengths and risk that are operating within the family system by implementing both of these tools together in the same assessment. This review is best done prior to a stressful life event that has the potential to destabilize the family and there are few that have such potential as the deployment of a family member.

The genogram is a powerful assessment tool that has been used for decades in the social science fields to identify intergenerational patterns of adaptation to stress that have emerged over time and place. The guiding principles for developing a resilience-based genogram include that all families, individuals, and communities have the inherent capacity to transform themselves and change the narrative of their lives and this can be facilitated by identifying and affirming the strengths of family and peer environments (Walsh, 2016). This resilience-oriented approach does not ignore family problems but rather it normalizes a family's distress and identifies the family's strengths to manage that distress through collaborative problem-solving strategies. The process of co-constructing a genogram with family members is therapeutic in that it helps to facilitate understanding of behaviors that developed as coping responses to problems in the past as well as the ways in which the family tends to function as an interactional system. Genograms provide individual family members with valuable information and insights about the generations that came before them by filling in the known and unknown gaps of their family's history over the course of time. In developing resilience-based genograms, families learn about their relationships from an objective perspective that can assist them in identifying which coping strategies worked best for them in the past and be able to manage stressful situations in the present as a result of this process. The goals for resilience-oriented genograms include increasing the positive, prosocial connections within a family's network of relationships, and identifying relationships that encourage positive youth identity development, emotional support, and effective problem solving in times of stress.

The military genogram is a specific resilience-oriented genogram that utilizes the strengths-based perspective for increasing resiliency with military-connected communities that offers a unique perspective of the ways in which military service may have influenced family functioning throughout several generations (Weiss et al., 2010). As the military culture is focused on building upon strengths to overcome obstacles and achieve solutions to problems, the military genogram takes a solution-focused perspective and approach for building resiliency in service members and their families. The military genogram is also culturally sensitive to allow for both the risk and protective factors of being connected to the military to emerge in the process of creating it. The common set of shared values, traditions, worldviews, and expectations that are associated with the functioning of the family are highlighted throughout its creation. Military families approach problems within the larger context of the military umbrella and this shapes a family's perceptions about challenges that are critical to learn when utilizing the military genogram's solution-focused approach for resiliency building with military families (Weiss et al., 2010). This military umbrella encompasses the risk and protective factors (strengths and weaknesses) inherent in the military family lifestyle to understand military family resiliency.

The military currently operates in the spheres of land, water, air, and space in terms of a total defense force with multiple branches and ways of serving from active duty to reserves to National Guard units. Despite these differences, there are unifying values, customs, and codes for behaviors that are shared across the branches. Military core values are the strengths that guide behavior and are required as part of the military culture from the initial indoctrination into the organization's belief system. Military ethos upholds the following values: courage, honor, loyalty, integrity, commitment, being fit for duty, the military missions being the priority for service members over self and family needs, and the concept of unit cohesion over individual needs or wants (Exum, Coll, & Weiss, 2010; Weiss et al., 2010).

The many traditions, customs, and ceremonies is another area to include in military genograms for discussions around resiliency in terms of points in time that may have been significant in military family life such as the traditions of promotion ceremonies for service members. Military service members have significant markers or points in time in their military careers that are celebrated and recognized publicly as they attain higher ranks that have significant impact on family life. While promotions often bring increased salary for a military family, they are often associated with increased responsibilities and commitment to the military as a result. Direct and honest conversations with family members around the meaning that such promotions hold for family life are important and add to increased understanding of the family's history in terms of how the military impacts family life. In addition to the influence of the service member's military careers on family life, a military genogram would also identify the role that any informal traditions have on family life such as the presence of alcohol in social gatherings with and without family members. A review of this aspect of military life may raise other related issues as part of the discussion and increase understanding of family adaptation to stress in doing so. Family members may discover an intergenerational pattern of coping behaviors with alcohol or other substances and in doing so determine possible points where its use as a coping strategy may have transformed from being adaptive to maladaptive and enhance understanding of potential reasons for this transformation. In discussions such as these, cultural traditions and norms are discussed and understood in concrete ways for their impact on family life and family adaptation to stress. The process of co-constructing a military family genogram would also include coping and adaptation responses following wartime military service across several generations and the ways in which family members managed these times especially if there were injuries or stress that lingered in the family (Weiss et al., 2010).

The military value of strength and the importance of being physically and mentally fit is a cultural norm in military life that translates into the often daily use of exercise to maintain levels of fitness necessary for military duty. The use of exercise and strength training among military personnel is another shared custom that is also commonly used as a cultural coping strategy for managing stress. Military service members and/or veterans who sustain physical injuries that take an extended time to heal or become chronic and persistent impairments in daily life may be at heightened risk for adaptive coping. If one's primary coping strategy is the use of exercise to relieve stress and manage difficult situations or emotions, the presence of physical injury needs to be assessed in terms of how long it will last and what other coping strategies might be employed during this period of time. Military-connected individuals who may be injured and unable to exercise may be at risk for maladaptive coping strategies to relieve stress, manage emotions, and take the place of an exercise regime. In the process of making behavioral choices for stress management, the military culture being one that is steeped in rigidity and fixed patterns for behaviors at every point in military life does not lend itself well to the flexibility hallmark of resiliency. In the process of making behavioral choices for stress management, the notion that flexibility in one's thinking can be highly adaptive and advantageous to achieving one's goals can be developed as a prevention strategy to respond well to setbacks such as injuries. In this manner, coping strategies are reviewed for their effectiveness as they may not provide the same degree of stress management that was achieved for that person in previous situations. In this way, rigid patterns of thinking would be encouraged to become less rigid and more flexible to problem-solve alternate solutions as coping responses. Discussions around core values may be helpful in generating new and more flexible responses for military family members who are not accustomed to utilizing flexibility in patterned responses to stress. Cognitive flexibility is problem solving how a family wants to live according to their core values while adapting to a new situation allows for new solutions to emerge and resiliency to flourish as a result. Some key areas to include in designing questions for a military-focused family genogram are included in the Appendix.

Measuring Resiliency: The Military Family Timeline

The Military Family Timeline is another useful assessment tool that is co-created among family members and different than an individual's timeline which begins at birth; the family timeline begins when the couple/parents first met. The family timeline is a visual depiction of the family's history and includes family crises, celebrations, deployments, health/mental health concerns, deaths, and other significant life events. Questions to consider include: "How did you cope with the crisis and what worked? What were major obstacles at the time? Is there anything you wish you had done differently to manage a stressful situation or to better celebrate a life event?" The timeline identifies the core family values and challenges the family narrative to consider what information might be missing in that narrative. Family members become aware of conflicting stories, diverse perceptions of blame and responsibility for major life situations, and actions taken by members to manage and adapt at the time.

The timeline offers families a chance to look at older stories through the lens of time and make connections as to how crises shaped the family narrative and what needs to shift to become a unified and cohesive story that the family can carry with them in the present challenge and into future stressful situations. A cohesive family narrative that is shared among all members makes families more resilient as they come to perceive that they are not alone in stressful times and can turn to others for support to navigate the challenges. A family's core values can be woven into this narrative to foster a shared sense of identity and sense of belonging to the family. Families can consider naming three of their most important values that are shared with all members in the family. In a light-hearted manner, family members can be asked to co-create their "Family Bumper Sticker" that could be put on the family car to tell the whole world just who they are as a family. Some examples of these mottos include: "We Never Stop; You're Never Alone with the Kodas; There's Always Room for One More; or Running Just as Fast as We Can!"

Measuring Resiliency: The Family Assessment

The Walsh Family Resilience Questionnaire contains 32 questions that family members answer on a scale from 1 to 5 and can help to establish a baseline understanding of a family's overall functional ability to respond in healthy ways to stressful situations (Walsh, 2016). Statements such as "We can share positive feelings, appreciation, humor, and fun and find relief from difficulties (p. 358)" will assess a family's ability to experience a wide range of emotions which is a crucial skill when managing high levels of distress in a family. Families who may need to manage posttraumatic stress in the future are especially vulnerable to having their emotional world become constricted to negative affective states as a result of such stress. Military families who are preparing for the possibility of a service member going to war would be protecting themselves from future complications in the event that any posttraumatic stress lingers or is unresolved in the family system following the return. In this way, families of veterans benefit from the educational awareness that a restricted range of affect is a symptom that needs to be balanced with the adaptive coping strategy of shared laughter and a sense of humor. Families who experience high levels of traumatic stress are at risk for the associated complications from it such as cognitive perceptions of the world being a dangerous place to live that can easily lead to maladaptive behavioral reactions to this belief and various levels of depression. One small question that assesses positivity in the family system can open up an entire dialog around coping strategies and educate families about the importance of humor and lightness to counteract potentially pervasive negativity that could permeate a family in times of great difficulty and distress.

Since there are 32 such questions in the Walsh Family Resilience Questionnaire, and each one holds the opportunity to educate family members on potential areas of vulnerability to stress, this assessment tool can be woven throughout multiple meetings with families (Walsh, 2016). Another question that is valuable in the process of establishing a family's strengths and potential areas of risk or vulnerability is: "We approach a crisis as a challenge we can manage and master with shared efforts (p. 357)." This statement not only assesses the family's ability to unify in times of stress but it also educates the family about how to identify when a situation is a crisis and how that family defines the idea of what a crisis looks like for them. This conversation opens up how the family has managed crises in the past, which will let them know what works for them in a solution-focused approach that identifies and names an adaptive coping strategy that they can employ again in the future. In addition to this coping strategy, families in crisis sometimes aren't aware that they are in crisis, and identifying what a crisis would look like for their family is important information for planning purposes. While some families may identify behavioral "red flags" as pointing to the presence of a crisis situation, other families may label a depletion in resources available to meet the demands of the situation. Resources may include a breakdown in informal support networks such as extended family or it can include depleted financial resources, limited childcare, and a spouse needing to work outside the home in paid employment. As mental health workers working with families who may be in crisis, it is valuable information to know especially because a provider's definition of a family crisis may be vastly different than any particular family's definition. It is crucial to establish whether these definitions are aligned and if not, where they diverge, because one person's crisis may be viewed as another person's challenge, and these perceptions are critical to establish. In this way, perception of problem or situation will be key components in shaping behaviors and beliefs about strength and vulnerability.

As this questionnaire can take several meetings to complete with the educational component that is possible with each answer, this assessment tool can also be offered in group settings such as to multi-family groups, groups of adolescents or spouses, and in the military setting through behavioral health providers under Medical Command. Groups such as these would be preventative in nature and designed to assist individuals and families in becoming aware of the different areas of functioning that they may excel in and the ones they could benefit from improving in certain ways. The process of completing such an assessment tool would strengthen a family's overall level of resilience to stress which is crucial for military families facing constant demands and changing stressful situations.

Building Community Capacity to Manage Stress

The perceptions of social or neighborhood cohesion, often defined as the extent to which neighbors trust and count on one another, has been demonstrated to serve as a buffer for individuals and protect them against stress and negative mental health effects. In studies ranging from the mental health benefits of social support for veterans, to individuals struggling with mental health conditions, and to depression from social isolation and loneliness, the perception that one has other people to rely on who support their experiences is a key component in resiliency (Robinette et al., 2021; Ruiz, Scholes, & Bobak, 2018). Individuals and families that perceive their social networks, neighborhoods, and communities as cohesive tend to perceive stressful situations as being less stressful and have better emotional and behavioral adaptations as a result. One study found that the greater the level of neighborhood cohesion, the lower the effect that posttraumatic stress had on parenting, in terms of certain challenges and difficulties in these roles (Franz et al., 2022).

The global pandemic of 2020 caused daily life to become confined to families, small groups of people, and neighborhood communities and led research studies to examine the effects of social networks on resiliency in the general population that had been mostly theoretical prior to the pandemic. The pandemic resulted in drastic increases in time spent with family, at home, and in one's neighborhood or community and positive perceptions of those environments were influential in terms of resiliency, mental health, and overall psychosocial wellbeing (Robinette et al., 2021). Neighborhoods where individual members perceived a sense of neighborhood cohesion during the pandemic and had social relationships that involved an exchange of community resources had a higher degree of trust and accountability than neighborhoods lacking such perceptions between members. The pandemic study reported that people perceiving more cohesion in their neighborhoods were more resilient in terms of mental health during the pandemic than individuals lacking perceptions of neighborhood or social cohesion. This finding in the general population supports the military ethos regarding the benefits that accompany perceptions of social cohesion among military service members and military communities and that this cohesion is a protective buffer against stress that can increase mental health resiliency for individuals and families.

The strength of one's social networks has power to support individuals and families through the most difficult and challenging times through formal and informal ways. These networks have been called "social capital" to reflect the resource inherent in social networks that can be as useful as financial capital if harnessed and utilized to its potential (Putnam, 2015). Putnam's ongoing work cautions that communities in the United States are in danger due to an erosion in social capital from reduced social interactions among individuals necessary for communities to thrive through the power of collective action. Similar to the way that financial resources (capital) can be invested and grow over time, social and community resources through civic engagement and relationships are investments in building a community that can support and sustain individual members. The idea that individuals are never as strong as groups provides the foundation for understanding the benefits that can be developed for future times when important resources may need to be utilized and called into action. Strength that is located in one's social networks through the acts of civic engagement is referred to as community capital. The combination of formal and informal networks both within and outside the military environment form the cornerstone for building community capacity for military families. Building networks between military and civilian resources often leads to the accrual of social capital and a mutual environment of support for military families (Huebner et al., 2009). The result of building community capacity is that a network of support is created that serves as a protective buffer against stress that leads to healthy family adaptation, community satisfaction, and overall well-being (Mancini, Martin, & Bowen, 2003). Veterans following wartime deployments often report that individual forms of support were not as important as the overall sense of community and that formal and informal supports were less significant than the perception of being a significant contributing member of one's community (Bobrow et al., 2013).

Part 2

Deployment Resiliency

"Managing the Storm"

4 Military Families Adapting to Stress

Role Exit Theory

During a deployment, military family members need to adapt to and tolerate many uncomfortable feelings, including that there are days when family members do not know where the service member is geographically, or the risk level involved on a daily basis. Feelings such as anxiety, confusion, powerlessness, and grief are some of the more common responses in terms of what families tolerate in family resiliency and adaptation to stress. Resilient families employ adaptive coping skills that build up their supply of resources and protective factors such as creating social networks, maintaining a sense of optimism for the future, staying physically healthy, and strengthening community ties to both formal and informal networks. Some of the more common maladaptive coping responses include emotional distancing, addiction, infidelity, reckless or self-destructive behaviors, staying busy to avoid feelings, avoiding social situations, isolating, and being less involved in one's community. Mental health symptoms that emerge in times of overwhelming stress are often a result of a depleted supply of resources available to meet the needs and demands of the stressful situation. Military family members living through a deployment situation are at risk for becoming overwhelmed due to the combination of factors including situational events in the family, the supply of resources available, and the perceptions of threat held by individual family members to health and safety. The absence of the service member, the ever-present threat of death, the additional role responsibilities and changes in the family system, depletions in resiliency levels among individual family members, and daily demands from life circumstances all combine and present risk to the family system. When coping strategies are not effective at managing the stressful situation that arises for a family during a deployment, mental health and overall functioning can deteriorate, and the demands far outweigh the system's ability to manage them effectively.

> *"I could see the reactions in my fellow service members immediately after phone calls with family members at home ended. It didn't matter if they received good news or bad news from their families back home, either way they would all walk away from the call looking upset, lonely, isolated, sad, angry, whatever emotions came up, you could see it clearly at that point. You never saw it as clearly as it was at that moment when they were leaving the call center on a deployment. They missed their families. We all did. Every communication with home caused us to remember them and the reminders of what we were missing: birthdays, football games, graduations, skinned knees, even minor events like falling off a bicycle could shake someone up because the little things were the reason we were there in the first place and the motivation that kept us going on most days.*

DOI: 10.4324/9781003438229-7

> *We were risking our lives for those little things and the freedoms that come with being a civilian and the civilian way of life that so many generations before us fought to preserve. So yes, those little stories that probably seemed so insignificant to our families back home were so important to hear even though it could be hard on us. We had to put all of those feelings somewhere safe to protect them. Once we had time to walk away from the call center, and get out of that headspace, we were back to normal but for that minute or two you could see everyone's feelings. They were on their faces and in the way they walked with their shoulders dropped and their eyes focused anywhere they could find to distract themselves. I once even thought it would be better to cut off all communication with our families back home while we were on a deployment and then realized that would never be the right thing to do. The possibility of us dying was real and every conversation had to be positive because it might be the last one they carried with them for the rest of their lives."*

Role exits happen throughout all of our lives, sometimes a result of a joyous, happy occasion such as marriage or adopting a child, and sometimes happening when a situation is not working out as in a career change or a marriage that ends in divorce. Role Exit Theory was described by Helen Rose Fuchs Ebaugh following her personal departure from the role of being a Catholic nun to that of wife, mother, and professor of sociology. She describes the process of "role exit" as being the departure from a role that was central to one's identity and encompasses specific stages that are based on disengagement, dis-identification, and re-socialization (Ebaugh, 1988). The four stages of leaving a role and constructing a new role, with a new identity that incorporates that new role, are as follows: (1) First Doubts: an individual experiences doubts or uncertainty about a current role they are living; (2) Seeking Alternatives: the individual looks outside of the current role to other roles; (3) Turning Points: events or behaviors trigger a decision to leave the current role; and (4) Creating the Ex-Role: a new identity is created through a new role. This theory was later applied to military couples experiencing marital conflict following a military deployment in a small, qualitative study where all of the couples had described a strong marital relationship prior to the deployment (Gambardella, 2008). For almost half of the couples, the at-home spouses were not able to exit the roles they had moved into during the deployment, specifically the role of independence. It appeared that for these spouses, the "role-exit" from dependency or inter-dependency in the marriage to having taken on new tasks, learned new skills, and gained independence was not an exit they wanted to make. For these spouses, the sense of mastery and competency that they achieved as a result of the demands of the military, left them without the doubt or uncertainty that was required to exit the new role that had developed in the absence of the service member.

Feelings of independence, mastery, competency, and confidence that arise as a result of role changes during deployments can offer military couples and families some relief from the more challenging and painful feelings that come with the deployment experience. The ever-present risk of serious injury and death that is associated with combat deployments typically generates overwhelming feelings of anxiety and stress for military families. The difficult feelings that arise from these deployment separations range from anxiety to sadness and depression if the separation is experienced as an abandonment and require all family members to find ways to manage these feelings to keep the family functioning. There are many internal and outward behavioral responses generated among and between family members to manage higher-risk deployment situations. Military families were often able to tolerate the "high-operational tempo" of the military during the post-9/11 wars by balancing the losses with gains achieved during the separations. Military couples were often able to tolerate marital conflict that stemmed from this dilemma because both partners knew that another separation or deployment was on the horizon for them. In this way, a second (or third, fourth, or fifth) long-term deployment separation signaled an exit from a family system that was operating with role confusion, doubt about stability, and uncertainty on a consistent basis and led to decreased resiliency. For both the military service member and the military spouse, the exit from role confusion in the family and re-entrance into role competency often helped families to manage and tolerate very difficult feelings surrounding wartime deployments. There is a great deal of research in the literature on the experiences of service members going to and returning home from war and how these experiences shape their perceptions, identities, and ways in which they see the world. There is far less research, however, on ways in which the deployment experience shapes the perceptions and identities of military spouses and children at home. If you were to ask military spouses and children how many people ever asked them how the deployment experience shaped their identities, worldviews, and their relationships, the answer will often be "none." As the conceptualization of family adaptation to stress relies heavily on the perceptions of all of the individual family members, it is crucial to understand the changes to the worldviews and self-perceptions surrounding identity for military families.

Military Adolescents at Risk

There exists a widespread concern about adolescent substance use in the general civilian population in the United States. Substance misuse can lead to problematic, and sometimes deadly, behaviors including transmission of sexually transmitted infections, deaths by car accidents, academic problems, unwanted pregnancies, juvenile delinquency, and risks to overall health and resiliency. Adolescents are particularly susceptible to involvement in substance misuse due to the developing state of the adolescent brain, which can involve reduced executive functioning, limited decision-making abilities, perceived infallibility, impulsivity, and increased risk for impairments in certain areas of cognitive functioning.

Serious risk factors that often contribute to the onset of substance use and misuse among adolescents fall into three categories: familial, social, and individual risk factors (Whitesell et al., 2013). Familial risk factors include childhood adverse experiences including maltreatment from abuse, neglect, and/or trauma; parental or familial substance abuse; interpersonal family violence; the quality of the parent–child relationships; and the adolescent perception that parents approve of substance misuse. Social factors that lead to increased risk for adolescent substance misuse include associating with a peer group who uses substances, which is often associated with conflictual (negative) parent–child relationships. Parental involvement in their children's lives, warmth, and mutual respect between parents and their teenagers is often associated with decreased maladaptive substance use (Whitesell et al., 2013). The research supports the notion and the significance of positive parent–child relationships being an important protective factor in terms of coping and adaptation. In addition to external risk factors for adolescent substance misuse/abuse, there are also individual factors that can contribute to the risk for being vulnerable to developing a substance use disorder. The use of alcohol and other substances during the period of adolescence is often a form of experimentation as some teens use substances to try out new behaviors and ways of interacting with others socially as part of forming an adult identity. Substance use in any stage of development can become maladaptive if it is a means for managing stressful situations and strong emotions that are intolerable or negative in any way. In military families, risk factors for adolescent misuse of alcohol and substances include longer parental deployments, frequent geographic relocations, disruptions in routines, and associated losses in terms of academic learning, achievement, and social connections (Blamey & Phillips, 2019). The findings support an earlier study with youth in Iowa that found that children of deployed military personnel in the Iowa National Guard and Reserves were at higher risk for alcohol and cannabis use compared with civilian children (Acion et al., 2013). The increase in substance use is likely due to the overlap of the parental deployment and a disadvantaged social situation as many of the children were living with someone other than a parent or relative at the time of the deployment. This group of children were from families of the National Guard and Reserve components and it would be interesting to find out if these results were similar to children living on military bases (active-duty families) with the added social support networks imbedded there and/or who lived with at least one parent during a parental deployment.

The misuse of alcohol and substances in adolescence is a maladaptive coping mechanism for managing difficult and painful feelings as well as symptoms of anxiety and depression. Depression often includes feelings of sadness, emotional pain, abandonment, loss, perceived rejection, isolation, powerlessness, hopelessness, despair, and anger. Depression may also result from familial stressors such as parental divorce, parental substance abuse, clinical depression of a family member, or feelings of inadequacy, which some adolescents report to be a motivating force for them to begin substance use in an attempt to feel better (Whitesell et al., 2013). These attempts to feel better are often referred to as coping through "self-medication" for adolescents who may not be diagnosed with depression but still suffer from it despite the lack of diagnosis and/or treatment.

Depression and substance use disorders often occur together in both adolescence and adulthood and one study found that depressed boys are 12 times more likely to become dependent on alcohol than boys without depression and depressed girls are four times more likely to become dependent on alcohol than girls without depression (Whitesell et al., 2013). Screening for depression and substance use would be beneficial to the military in terms of adolescent health, mental health, and overall family readiness as screening would allocate resources to assist youth in getting necessary therapeutic support to prevent and/or treat these co-occurring conditions. To strengthen youth and family resiliency during the deployment of a military parent, early identification of the risk factors for depression would improve the family's ability to prevent the maladaptive coping response of alcohol or substance misuse to emerge during a parental deployment.

In situations where a family member is experiencing episodes of destabilization, family life can escalate quickly into situations of heightened risk for interpersonal conflict and even physical altercations when there is no concrete plan for managing out-of-control emotional states. When alcohol use is a regular part of family life, as it is in many military traditions and ceremonies, the escalation to misuse and abuse of it can be devastating to family stability. Alcohol impairs cognitive functioning, which means that it makes it more difficult to problem-solve and to control anger and other emotional affective states. This decrease and impairment in cognitive functioning makes it more likely for an individual to misread a situation and to react impulsively based on cognitive distortions. While alcohol can serve to numb an individual's feelings and emotions, it also limits the ability to think and respond to situations and other people rationally. Alcohol use following trauma is a widespread and often a very common coping strategy to manage traumatic stress and the associated symptoms that follow trauma. Alcohol is often used to tolerate the heightened physiological states that accompany traumatic stress that are often described as a constant "adrenaline drip" that runs 24 hours/day every day. It also assists with the related symptoms, including: difficulty sleeping at night due to nightmares; to dull reactions to triggers and flashbacks (both internal and environmental); to increase sociability and counteract social avoidance; and to avoid negative memories, thoughts, and feelings related to the trauma. Two or more negative alterations in cognition and mood are diagnostic criteria found in the diagnosis of posttraumatic stress disorder as per the most recent American Psychiatric Association's Diagnostic Manual, the DSM-5 (APA, 2013). These criteria include pervasive negative beliefs about oneself, others, or the world not present prior to the trauma; distorted cognitions around responsibility for the traumatic events; persistent negative emotions and irritability; decreased interest/participation in activities; feelings of detachment from others; and a persistent inability to experience positive emotions. Although alcohol use provides a temporary sense of relief from overwhelming traumatic stress and may allow positive emotions to be experienced, it also impairs the ability to challenge problematic thoughts that fuel the stress and prevent it from being resolved.

The Double ABCX Theory of Family Adaptation to Stress

Family adaptation to stress has been the focus of generations of researchers who strove to understand the effects of wartime deployment stress on military families. These researchers studied how family adaptation depends on multiple factors including a family's resources, values, beliefs, and perceptions of whether or not they can meet the demands. The ABCX Theory was developed by Hill in 1949 to understand how military families managed in the midst of World War II, including how they adapted to the stress, and how they managed the crisis of wartime separation as a family. In the 1970s and 1980s, family researchers expanded on Hill's work to better understand the phases of adjustment that families went through as they adapted to the wartime crisis of service members who were missing in action in Vietnam. Researchers McCubbin and Patterson (1983) studied 216 families who were in crisis for years waiting for their family member to return home (an average of 6.6 years) and conceptualized a new model that accounted for adaptation to stress over time called the Double ABCX Theory. The process that these families in crisis went through (in perception and behaviors) in response to the crisis was described as the Family Adjustment and Adaptation Response (FAAR) by McCubbin and Patterson (1983). The FAAR process included the pile-up of stressors and demands on the family; the new and existing resources in the family and the community to meet the demands; modifying the definition of the problem by attaching a new meaning to it; and coping strategies used to create changes in the family structure to be able to adapt in positive ways.

In the Double ABCX Theory, the "A" refers to the stressor (such as a deployment); the "B" refers to the family's existing resources (such as formal and informal support networks); the "C" refers to the cognitions/perceptions of the situation; and the "X" refers to the outcome in terms of behavioral changes and role shifts in the family (see Figure 4.1). These adaptations represent a new crisis when instability in the family system is present as systems strive for balance, organization, and predictability in routines and family roles. Individuals and families make accommodations in the process of adjusting to stress to meet the demands of a very difficult situation and these can be resilient or problematic. During

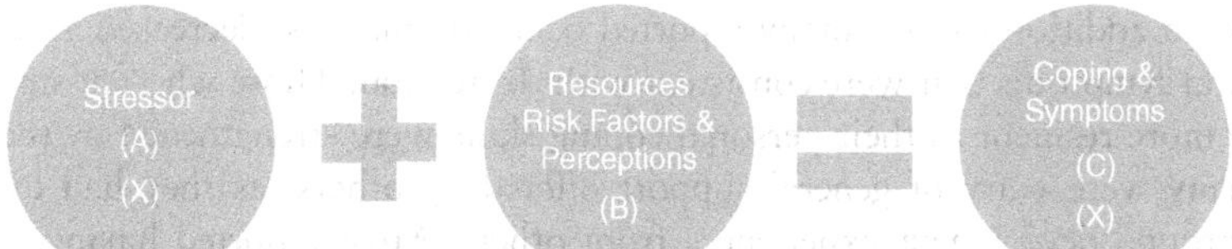

Figure 4.1 The double ABCX model of family adaptation to stress (McCubbin and Patterson, 1983)

the process of accommodating to change, healthy/adaptive coping and unhealthy/maladaptive coping strategies may result and can add to a family's resiliency or contribute to future problematic functioning. In situations of adaptation to stress, the construct of the intergenerational transmission of stress is important to highlight as families that have not had the resources or perceptions of being able to manage the demands of the situation may experience increased challenges over time due to complicated patterns of interactions within and outside the family.

Multiple variables determine when a given event becomes a crisis in a family and some of the most significant of these include the following: the significance of the event itself; the availability of resources that the family can access to meet the demands of the situation; clarity of the roles in the family; flexibility in the family's thinking and approaches to problem solving (trying new and creative ways to meet challenges if old ones do not work); and the family's overall perception of the event, including whether or not it was experienced as a threat to the family in any way. Family crises require changes in role performance as the family's usual patterns shift or disappear and the family needs to create new patterns for interacting with one another and the outside world based on these shifts. Crises generally emerge and become problematic in families when there is an unhealthy maladaptation to stressful situations, limited (or lack of utilizing) resources, and problematic perceptions regarding the magnitude and manageability of the problem.

The Double ABCX Theory is a theory of understanding how risk factors pile up and contribute to system overload based not only on the risk factors themselves, but also when these factors combine with the family's perceptions of the stress and their ability to manage risk factors. In this theory, a stressor can include a death in the family, a significant injury/illness or loss, or a significant separation for a family. The stressor is combined with the family's risk/protective factors and perception of manageability (positive or negative) of the stressor. These include the family's financial situation (strong, stable, or a current hardship), levels of education (higher levels are generally protective factors), ongoing strengths and challenges (previously established emotional stability or vulnerabilities/mental health challenges), existence or lack of social support networks, and other variables impacting the family's functioning. Research that was supported by the Military Family Research Institute and the DoD Quality of Life Office focused on adaptations that adolescents in military families make when a parent is deployed (Huebner & Mancini, 2005). Qualitative methods were used through focus groups conducted with youth attending camps in the summer of 2004 and found that many adolescents demonstrated great maturity during military deployments. These teens reported that they took on additional responsibilities at home, often referring to themselves as having become a "co-parent" for younger siblings, and that providing such additional support for the parent remaining at home was one of the most important tasks assumed and represented significant shifts in their roles, responsibilities, and emerging identities as a result. These adolescents reported ongoing attempts to protect the at-home parent and their siblings from experiencing negative emotions and heightened levels of stress as they were very aware of the dangers associated with the deployment and the ways their lives changed as a result of it. Many teens reported missing after-school activities because there was no one to drive them there and/or not having enough family income to sign up for them. In addition to this, many reported behavior changes, decreased academic performance, and symptoms that were consistent with depression. Those who felt supported by others were more resilient as their personal coping skills were strengthened by the support, although many were wary of general support offered by others, as they had experienced insincerity around deployment experiences from others. Most reported having contact (e-mail or phone) at least once a week, often multiple times a week with their deployed parent and relied heavily on that parent to provide them with accurate information about the war because they did not believe that the media reported war-related events accurately (Huebner & Mancini, 2005). Recommendations from this study included increasing awareness that adolescents in military families may not have reached a developmental level to adequately communicate or discuss their feelings during a deployment, and that some adolescents do not speak with anyone about their fears, concerns, or sadness. This awareness speaks to the importance of adolescents getting involved in social support networks outside the family with individuals who can role model stress management skills and provide positive experiences filled with laughter, fun, and lightness to balance deployment-related stress at home. Adolescents who are encouraged to participate in the full range of emotions during stressful situations learn that carving out time and space for positive experiences can offer an emotional respite and protection against depression.

The adolescent study on adaptation to stress confirmed the addition of social support to the "B" category of resources in the Double ABCX model with formal and informal support included in the Community Capacity-Building Practice Model (Bowen et al., 2003; Huebner & Mancini, 2005). The Community Capacity-Building Practice Model helps to understand the relationship between community-based social networks and military family adaptation to deployment-related stress. Building community capacity that can support military youth includes intentionally designed programs with ongoing and easily accessible social activities for adolescents so they have opportunities to step outside the family situation and develop social networks with peers and mentors. Programs that help teens develop effective networking skills with peers include learning how to communicate feelings directly and honestly and develop friendship bonds that can sustain them through challenging times. It is also crucial for adolescents to develop mentoring bonds with older teens and/or young adults who had experienced the deployment of a military parent for additional social support and role modeling. Formal support programs that encourage the development of informal networks of peers and peer mentors normalize the experience for military teens while offering them a sense of belonging, a distraction and respite from the stress at home, positive experiences, and hopefulness that they will adapt successfully to meet the demands of their challenging situation.

Characteristics of Resilient Families Adapting to Wartime Military Service Across History (Hill, 1949 to Present):

1. Previous success in managing and overcoming family crises;
2. Non-materialistic goals predominate family values;
3. Flexibility and willingness to shift traditional roles;
4. Acceptance of responsibility by all family members in duties;
5. Willingness to sacrifice personal interests for family objectives;
6. Pride in the family tree and intergenerational traditions;
7. Presence of strong patterns of emotional interdependence and unity;
8. High participation as a family in joint activities;
9. Presence of equal patterns of family control and decision-making;
10. Strong affectional ties (between parents, parents–children, children–children).

In addition to these characteristics of resilient families, Hill reported on the differences in communication styles among military families during wartime separation and described three different categories: closed ranks, open ranks, and partially closed ranks.

Families who operate as a closed system (closed ranks) are designed for intimacy to be kept within the family and behaviors typically exclude the outside world. This system often leads to feelings of smothering confinement for individual family members as well as the exclusion of the absent military parent during deployment separations. The families who had "closed ranks" lived their lives without interference from the deployed parent, who was considered as being outside of the family system during military service; there was little or no communication with that person, who had no input into family decision-making while away; the person's chair was either physically removed from the dining table or another person had occupied that person's chair during the separation (Hill, 1949). Families who employed "open ranks" to adapt to the military service member being away from home made great efforts to include the absent person with constant communication and ongoing decision-making involvement. These families were mentally keeping that person's place in the family system and would leave his or her chair at the table and unoccupied until the service member returned home. Families who utilized "partially closed ranks" would include the service member when deemed necessary for serious issues or incidents at home. In terms of how these families adjusted to loss of service members who were killed in the war, the families with open ranks had serious bereavement adjustments to make as they had kept that family member involved in the system at all times. The families with closed ranks had already made a systemic adjustment to the loss of the service member in the family's daily life and had less concrete changes to make as a result (Hill, 1949). It is almost as if the families who "closed ranks" were preparing for the worst should it happen and because of this, had made adjustments to life without the service member should their fears become reality. The families who lived with the service member as part of daily life psychologically lived with a sense of hopefulness about the future and with the expectation that the deployed parent would return home safely one day and resume their previous role in the family system.

Attachment Theory and Affect Management

> *"A way of conceptualizing the propensity of human beings to make strong affectional bonds to particular others, and of explaining the many forms of emotional distress and personality disturbance, including anxiety, anger, depression, and emotional detachment to which unwilling separation and loss give rise".*
>
> Bowlby, 1969

The family's attachment system allows families to manage stressful situations based on interactional patterns that are qualitatively described as adaptive, disengaged, enmeshed or a combination of these among family members. In a deployment situation, the family's sense of stability and security can become weak or compromised as a primary attachment figure, the military parent, becomes unavailable and the at-home caregiver as well as children, siblings, and parents fear for the safety of the service member. In addition to fearing for the military parent's safety, the family as a whole experiences an ongoing threat to the safety of the system as a result, and responds to that threat with heightened levels of attachment insecurity. The family as a system employs coping strategies to manage this insecurity and responds to the situation in either adaptive or maladaptive ways, based on previously established interactional patterns for managing stress. The concept of the internal working model that is formed in early childhood attachment relationships forms the templates for how individuals cope with stressful situations, regulate emotions, and interact in close relationships. Family members may respond to the stress of a deployment situation with themes of attachment avoidance through a denial of emotions or attachment anxiety that is evidenced through emotional ambivalence toward the absent service member.

Family members with histories of insecurity in their attachment bonds (including the parent–child, child–child, and adult–adult relationships) are at heightened risk in terms of their resiliency and responses to stressful situations. Individual family members with insecure attachment bonds are at risk when the system is not able to guarantee that their needs for safety and security will be met and this is especially true for children who are dependent on their system to meet all their physical and emotional needs. Individual family members without secure attachment relationships in the family system are likely to experience great difficulty managing strong affective states, become easily flooded and overwhelmed by their emotions, and emotionally dysregulated as a result. The risk factor of the traumatic situation of a loved one going to war complicates this process for family members without secure attachment histories, or those experiencing a disruption or loss of the internalized attachment figure from the separation, and they may become preoccupied with the dangerousness of the situation. Secure attachment bonds serve to promote affect regulation that helps to tolerate emotional threats to safety through the presence of soothing internalized relationship bonds from a sense of object constancy of that connection. The experience of a deployment can lead to overwhelming affective states that threaten a cohesive sense of self when object constancy is not experienced by individual family members, especially young children who may not have achieved this developmental milestone yet. Clinical treatment interventions that improve object constancy, strengthen family attachment bonds, and teach affect management skills can help in strengthening individual and family resiliency during the deployment situation.

The experience of going to war has profound effects on everyone in the family and communication can be difficult especially at times when service members are required to limit communication with family members about events they are experiencing on a daily basis. The limiting of communication may be due to reasons of operational security, to keep family members safe by not knowing too many details of a mission, and in cases of the death of a service member on a unit's deployment when the immediate family has not been informed. The overall effect of shutting down family communication, however, is that it raises anxiety levels because the family does not have information about what is happening and many family members have to make intentional efforts not to jump to negative conclusions or catastrophic thinking during these times. At other times, the quality of communication can break down during a deployment and become limited or superficial as family members respond dynamically to one another in conversations, especially times when information might be vague or left out, as often happens on the part of the service member who may be reluctant to share certain details that are negative with family members. Families who fall into a pattern of not sharing information and do not explain the reasons why they are limiting content in communications, are at risk for not knowing how to shift away from this in the post-deployment phase. There are several responses that can arise in response to significant decreases in the quality and quantity of information being shared from changes in behavioral patterns to increased confusion or distressed emotions. Family members may experience feeling a loss of control over their ability to manage their emotions and internal affects as a result of limits in communication, especially families who are highly communicative and share emotions openly as a means of understanding them and making meaning out of them in daily life.

Navigating Ambiguous Loss in the Military Family

How one manages ambiguous loss in relationships is highly influenced by attachment styles and is one of the most powerful processes in family life able to reactivate insecure attachment patterns that may have been dormant for years among family members. Individual family members with previous histories of insecurity in their attachments with primary childhood caregivers are at heightened risk in terms of resiliency due to this insecurity during times of extended physical separations from loved ones. In addition to physical separations, families experiencing ambiguous loss are at heightened risk for attachment insecurities to arise that can easily compromise the process of healthy adaption to stressful situations. Attachment insecurities that go unrecognized and not addressed between family members can lead to behaviors that are maladaptive for individuals and unproductive to the overall functioning of the family system as a whole. The activation of an insecure attachment pattern in a family threatens the stability of the family as a secure base for emotional safety and places members at risk for mental health symptoms to develop as a result. An insecure attachment pattern that becomes activated in response to a stressful situation and leads to significant changes in behaviors among family members may also cause members to draw conclusions that may not be accurate perceptions of the problem. In the presence of misinterpretations, and cognitive distortions of the situation, family members will need corrective information about the experience to be able to return to a sense of stability.

The concept of ambiguous loss emerges during the absence of the service member in the family system during a deployment separation as that person's roles and responsibilities in the family become distributed to the family members at home. Families that deny the ambiguous loss are at risk for not managing the separation well or for being resilient. Ambiguous loss in a family system occurs when one member is physically absent and emotionally present, or physically present and emotionally absent. In other words, that family member is "gone but not gone" or "here but not here" in terms of the effects and impact of the loss on the family system (Boss, 2009). Boss points out that many people do not emotionally disconnect, disengage, or detach from loved ones just because they are physically absent and at the other extreme do not always emotionally connect with family members who are present in their lives. Families typically include those members with periodic or gradually deteriorating cognitive/emotional abilities and attachments and encourages using the term "psychological family" to address these qualitative nuances and sense of belonging. Members of our psychological family may include those who are with us physically but not able to interact with us, such as family members experiencing dementia, brain injury, addiction, depression, and other chronic illnesses as well as military service members on deployments or missing in action (Boss, 2009).

The Impact of Boundary Ambiguity on Resiliency

Boundaries in families include both physical and psychological processes that foster a sense of group and individual identity that differentiates the members of a family from one another and from other groups (Boss, 2009). Boundary ambiguity in families is a state in which family members are unclear in their perceptions about who is in or out of the family and who is performing what roles and tasks within the family system (Boss, 2009). An example of boundary ambiguity that often comes up in family therapy occurs when a couple who have children get divorced from one another but remain in their parenting roles, keep in regular communication, and attend events such as holidays, children's sports, birthday parties, graduations, and other social events despite being divorced.

Their roles as spouses to each other have ended in an actual, documented loss with a finality pronounced in court by a judge on a specific date with an exact time, but their roles as parents and in extended family relationships have changed in unclear, undefined ways that often lead to family boundary ambiguity.

Ambiguous loss is the most stressful kind of loss because it creates long-term confusion about who is in and who is out of a relationship or a family (Boss, 2009). Loss that is ambiguous in nature requires that family members have the capacity to hold contradictory views simultaneously, which is very difficult for some members to do, especially those in certain stages of child development, and those who have unresolved traumas from childhood that result in personality disorders that make holding opposing relational perceptions extremely difficult. Childhood trauma that goes unresolved can become entrenched into one's personality and make it nearly impossible to hold dialectically opposing views and perceptions simultaneously (such as happiness and sadness; good and evil). In addition to this difficulty, childhood trauma tends to lead to the creation of certain patterns of thinking that are cognitive distortions of self, others, and the world as being a safe and benign place in general. In the presence of ambiguous loss and boundary ambiguity in military families, trauma exposures need to be factored into the Double ABCX process of family stress management, as patterns of thinking and personality traits can impact an entire family's perspective and shape the family narrative making it very confusing for everyone in the family. In addition to trauma exposures, the presence of unresolved traumatic stress that is chronic and/or from childhood for one or both of the parents can impact parenting choices, styles of attachment bonding, and behaviors in the parent–child relationship that will impact the child's psychological and social–emotional development.

Ambiguous loss theory explains that the loss is different than a clearly defined loss such as death that has an official death certificate with the date, time of the death, and reason for what is a final and permanent loss of a family member. In addition to these clear and defined steps taken acknowledging a death, there are also clear rituals in the family and wider community that honor its occurrence and offer solace and comfort to the grief-stricken family (Boss, 2009). When there is no agreed-upon recognition of the loss, there is also no discussion of how to define the loss that can become problematic for families when boundary ambiguity is also present (confused ideas/perceptions of who is in or out of the family, who does what tasks, and who performs which roles in the family). This confusion can lead to feelings of hopelessness and prevent the family from being able to manage the stressful situation in ways that would be adaptive in nature that would otherwise allow the family to grieve the loss (Boss, 2009). These problems become new stressors that are then added onto the family's already burdensome situation and prevent the family from adapting to the stress and loss in healthy ways. Family members in these situations may be confused about how the family system works and who assumes which roles in the presence of boundary ambiguity.

Boundary ambiguity can result from two very different situations: one in which the facts surrounding the event are unclear or one in which the facts surrounding the event are clear, but for some reason, the family ignores or denies these facts (Boss, 2002). In such situations, the family holds a problematic perception that is different from that of an objective outside person. When an outside observer such as a family friend, a child's teacher, a community leader, spiritual leader, or mental health professional notices that their perception is very different from a family member's perception, the presence of boundary ambiguity should be considered as a possible contributing factor in the resolution of a family problem or a complicated grief process. Due to the fact that ambiguous loss is situated in the loss of a loved one in a relationship, the most effective treatment for understanding it and making meaning out of the confusion is through either family-based therapy or community-based social-supportive interventions rather than individual therapy (Boss, 2009).

Families need to be able to make sense of the new situation to be able to effectively adapt to it and create new family narratives with reorganized roles, tasks, and responsibilities. Children who are living in families experiencing situations of ambiguous loss with boundary ambiguity need developmentally appropriate explanations to understand the shifting family dynamics. When children understand their family's situation, they are able to create their own individual child-focused narratives. If these child-focused narratives are respected by the adult members and allowed expression in the larger family narrative, children will have increased feelings of confidence and mastery of the situation which will encourage them to seek out opportunities to repeat this process in future situations, with and without stress. In addition to these feelings that foster resiliency for the children in the family, these young family members will be given the experience of learning what healthy boundaries look like and feel like in a family.

Family narratives that are co-created among family members lead to greater understanding of changes in family functioning, daily interactions, and relationships in the family. A family that is able to create a coherent and logically consistent narrative to explain boundary ambiguity in the family system will be better equipped to perceive the situation as manageable. In light of this perception, daily problems then come with solutions shared with all members understanding what is going on as well as why and how stress is being managed. Behaviors that reflect both individual and group competency are able to develop through feelings of a sense of belonging and united family cohesiveness. The grieving process takes on a clear path forward that incorporates changes in family roles and relationships and new roles are charted with excitement and hopefulness toward the future.

The physical absence of the service member process places extra demands on the family system, and in order to maintain its functional capacity and equilibrium, the family needs to reorganize and redistribute the roles of the missing family member. The uncertainty of ambiguous loss can prevent a family from reorganizing roles because the family member is scheduled to return in a set timeframe. In military families, reorganizing to adjust to the loss of the service member gone to war is often experienced as overwhelming given the ever-present reality of possible death of the missing service member. A temporary redistribution of roles can be perceived as too threatening because of the reality that it could easily be a permanent shift in the family system. As a response to this perceived threat, a military family might cope with this loss through the use of denial of the grief and related feelings that are involved and as such will not redistribute roles and responsibilities.

The system will become frozen in place due to the confusion and unresolved grief and the family will become less able to meet the needs of individual family members as a result. When a family system functions at reduced capacity, it cannot provide the security that resilient families rely on to manage stressful events, and attachment insecurity can re-emerge for the adults and develop for the children. A family system that cannot provide a sense of safety and attachment security among family members is at heightened risk for reduced capacity for effective coping and management of strong affective states. In response to reduced stability and safety in a family, mental health symptoms are likely to develop and these often include: anxiety, depression, chronic headaches, fatigue and loss of interest/motivation, self-harming behaviors, substance misuse, disordered eating, and difficulty sleeping.

Children Living with Ambiguous Loss and Boundary Ambiguity

The impact of growing up in a family that is experiencing a loss that is ambiguous in nature is significant when there are no words or explanations used to describe the experience. The loss of a loved one's emotional or cognitive presence in daily life is an extremely confusing experience for adults to understand and even more so for children who are in developmental stages of concrete ways of thinking. Children will typically search for reasons to explain the change in the relationship and in their attachment to that person that is experienced as different and altered as a result. In the absence of explanations from adults in their lives, children are likely to experience anxiety and confusion until they find causality for the change and may even attribute the cause for it to themselves or recent behaviors on their part. In the case of military families experiencing deployment of a family member, a child left on his or her own to make sense of the situation might reach the conclusion that their behaviors caused the military service member to leave physically, or withdraw emotionally, from family members before or after the deployment situation. In families experiencing the emotional withdrawal of one or more family members that is inexplicable and unnamed, the attachment bond will be challenged due to the withdrawal. The withdrawal and resulting loss of emotional attachment will be a major source of stress in the child's life but the child's perception and understanding are equally important in terms of adaptation and resiliency outcomes.

Parenting Challenges (Case Example)

A military parent in a dual-military couple described one of the greatest challenges he experienced in parenting was due in part to his military training. While both parents were on separate deployments, their 14-year-old son lived with his maternal grandmother, and became depressed as he experienced great sadness with the loss of these significant relationships as well as the daily routines and rituals the three shared together in his daily life. When he returned home, his son was quick to anger, oppositional, and defiant with him and his grandmother. The service member's immediate response was to initiate what he called "an escalation of force" as he reportedly had learned in his tactical warfare training to overpower a potential threat to safety in the environment. Although he knew that his response was not working, he believed it was a problem residing solely within his son and not in the relationship between them, and took him to therapy to fix his son's problem. It came as a surprise to him that his son was experiencing depression since he left for his deployment shortly after his spouse had left and that his son's anger was due to his feelings of loss and powerlessness over the situation. The escalation of force did not create safety but rather it had the opposite effect of making everyone feel less safe as a result. He was relieved when he was able to talk about this with his son and listen to his son's experience of missing him during the deployment in a calm and reassuring manner. The creation of a well thought-out and planned response to his son's anger and out-of-control emotional states at home provided him with a "response prevention" for managing his reactions and achieving their mutual goal of stability in their home and in their relationship. He was able to shift his response when his son displayed oppositional and defiant behaviors around him and reassure him that their relationship was strong even though he did have to leave periodically for military assignments. It made sense to him from his military training that staying calm was effective in these situations to counteract his son's out-of-control emotional states and keep the family safe and functioning. The ability for father and son to open up their communication and to be direct and honest with each other about their feelings was the reason that they were able to adapt to the situation and find solutions to the problem. In this new way of communicating, they were able to identify that the son had become depressed due to worrying that his parents would never return and insecure about their family's future whenever either parent had to leave for trainings or deployments. They agreed to take steps to strengthen their attachment bond and together they collaboratively problem solved and came up with actions they could take during these separations to increase their reminders of one another. They took pictures together and printed them out, sent copies to the other parent, and chose one that they would keep with them at all times during family separations. They agreed to write to each other in a journal every night about their days, even if just one sentence, and compare these after the separations. Daily reminders increased their sense of security in their relationship and feelings of hopefulness that both were thinking of the other when they were apart which helped the son feel less depressed and he experienced less anger and more positive feelings overall in his daily life as a result.

5 Attachment Disruptions and Coping Strategies

Military Spouses and Civilian Careers

Civilian military spouses and children are dependents on the military organization, entitled to family support benefits and access to military installations. They typically accommodate to the military's needs in order to accompany the service member relocating geographically every time the military service member moves. Identification cards are necessary for entering onto bases and for government-sponsored facilities including gyms and pools, shopping for essential items like groceries, and to purchase household goods such as appliances and electronics, without paying state taxes of the location. Military families endure long periods of separation from one another during military deployments as well as regular trainings away from home still referred to as "yonder" in the acronym TDY, which stands for "temporary duty yonder." These periods require the military spouse at home to take on additional responsibilities, tasks, and roles that are otherwise filled by the service member in the family. In addition to these added responsibilities, active-duty military spouses typically assume many of the tasks involved in the repeated geographic relocations, all of which add up to make working outside of the home very difficult and career paths severely truncated. Despite often having more education than their civilian peers, military spouses have less income or earnings and are less likely to advance in their chosen careers as a result of multiple factors including regularly moving, taking on and letting go of additional role responsibilities, and sometimes deployment-related injuries to the service member that impact the entire family's functioning as a system. Reports estimate that less than half of all active-duty civilian spouses are in paid employment outside the home and of those spouses, only 60% work full-time (Meadows et al., 2016).

Many military spouses have higher rates of unemployment, underemployment, and lower wages than their civilian peers, which many attribute to the constant geographic relocations that interrupt spousal career paths and income trajectories. The military family in the current era of the all-volunteer force has become increasingly more of an integral part of active-duty life because more service members are getting married and having children and remaining in service longer than in previous generations. Although the military has always provided assistance and basic housing needs to military families, it has recently included programs aimed at supporting family resiliency and well-being such as subsidized, affordable early childhood family day care. This programmatic shift reflected the response to the increased numbers of families that emerged in the era of the all-volunteer force.

The career trajectories of active-duty military (civilian) spouses often do not follow a linear path because of the many geographic relocations and additional role responsibilities taken on in the family due to military missions that are often unpredictable. These

DOI: 10.4324/9781003438229-8

combine to often cause employers to be reluctant to hire them for jobs that require large investments in training or require predictability in availability for the job. Compared to their civilian counterparts, more spouses of service members are unemployed (not employed in paid labor outside of the home); underemployed (working fewer hours than they would like in paid labor outside of the home); and earning less income overall (Hosek & MacDermid Wadsworth, 2013). These moves also occur in tandem with the demands of military duty including long and often unpredictable working hours when the service member is at home and repeated deployments for extended periods away from home. This aspect of the military lifestyle requires that the spouses of service members have flexibility in their work schedules, particularly if there are children in the family who need routine care or have disabilities that require a higher-level of involvement from a parent or guardian. This flexibility demand often negatively affects the earnings of spouses regardless of gender or if they are in a dual-military couple or not. A chronic requirement for flexibility in one's employment also tends to have an impact on the choice of careers that are open to military spouses as they would be restricted to careers that can respond to change and meet their needs for flexibility. Spouses of military service members are less likely to work while a service member is away on a deployment and the rate of unemployment climbs higher if there are young or multiple children in the home. These transitions in a family typically call for renegotiation among family members regarding previously defined roles, shared responsibilities, and division of labor within the family and home environment. Spousal participation in the labor force outside of the home typically falls several months prior to a deployment and does not rise again until several months after the service member returns home (Hosek & MacDermid Wadsworth, 2013).

Despite the increasing numbers of women serving in the military and civilian male spouses, the majority of military civilian spouses remain female, and take on the roles of single parent regularly and in an unpredictable fashion as needed from demands of the military. Military policy plays a role in shaping military family choices as marriage and parenthood provides higher off-base housing/moving allowances and full family health coverage in addition to on-base resources. Some active-duty benefits include quality day care subsidized by the federal government, sports and recreational programs that are free to all family members, access to educational tutoring services, and planned social activities offered for children, youth, and families. The active-duty military population is more likely to be married and less likely to become divorced while on active duty than their civilian counterparts. These majority-female spouses make continued sacrifices to the military lifestyle in terms of career paths and social development in the public sphere outside of the domestic home life in the military community. Due to the constant demands of the military for extended work duties and deployments of service members, military spouses assume the roles and work of the service member within the family at routine intervals. The additional roles that include childcare and running a household, and the extra layers of support required by children in times of stress during deployments, create extra labor that is not paid and rarely given recognition. As a result, military spouses sacrifice occupational lives filled with daily achievements and feelings of competency that come from paid employment outside of the home. In addition to this, paid labor outside of the home increases levels of esteem and self-confidence that are empowering for individuals, protective in managing anxiety and depression, increase resiliency to stress, and tend to lead to increased levels of overall satisfaction and well-being.

The flexibility demand and the many geographic moves that military families endure lead many spouses to advance in their educational careers because they are able to combine classes from multiple colleges and training/certification programs. Military wives are more likely to have a college education than their civilian counterparts with 84% having at least some college education; 25% having college degrees, and 10% having advanced degrees (Bradbard, Maury, & Armstrong, 2016). Military spouses are paid less, work fewer hours, are often unemployed or underemployed and in jobs that are inconsistent with their education or experience, and have gaps on their résumés as a result of the military lifestyle (Meadows et al., 2016). The overwhelming majority of active-duty military spouses have repeatedly reported that the military lifestyle has had a negative impact on their careers overall and that they had often experienced difficulty finding employment.

Approximately 22% of military spouses are overeducated for their occupations with 40% of them experiencing an occupational mismatch, compared with civilian counterparts who experience less than 10% of a mismatch to their educational levels (Lim & Schulker, 2010). The demands of the military and its impact on spouses can be seen in common themes found on the résumés of military spouses in that they are often organized differently than résumés of their non-military civilian counterparts. Military spouses tend to have résumés that are presented in functional, rather than chronological, order often with a great deal of volunteer work, and educational programs often do not match the amount of time typically expected to complete the programs. There are often gaps in employment and education as seen in the following ways: educational degree programs not completed and/or prolonged time spent in programs to complete them; attendance at multiple colleges and training programs; holding multiple degrees (often unrelated or loosely-connected); a history of unrelated jobs; employment that was unrelated to their educational background or level of education; more volunteer work rather than paid work; shorter durations and periods of time holding jobs; underemployment (part-time or temporary jobs held); certifications in lieu of degree-earning educational diplomas; periods of long-term unemployment; and unclear career trajectory advancement often lacking increased responsibilities or skills attained over time in their careers (Bradbard, Maury & Armstrong, 2016).

Geographic moves tend to lead to a significant decline in hours worked by military spouses (generally 4–5 hours/week decrease) and in one's labor-market status for military spouses who experience an average 10% drop in employment as a result of a geographic relocation (Cooke & Speirs, 2005). Since the majority of young military service members starting families are in the lower ranks and fall into the lowest pay grades, many young military families experience financial hardship/stress, difficulties paying bills, and keeping up with financial obligations. It is common to see credit companies setting up offices and marketing material offering loans to military families just outside of military installations in the United States to take advantage of this situation and charging very high annual percentage rates for repayment. Many military families receive welfare and food stamps due to income levels that often lead to issues of food insecurity for them. In contrast to their civilian counterparts who tend to begin having children once they are in careers for a few years, military couples tend to become parents at much younger ages, have more children overall, and have children of younger ages in the family within a few years of getting married. Military spouses of service members in the Navy are the most likely to be in the labor force and most likely to earn the most income among military spouses in the other branches. However, across all of the branches, military spouses are more likely than their civilian counterparts to fall in the bottom 30% of the distribution of all wage earners and less likely to be in the top 40% (Lim, Golinelli, & Cho, 2007).

The context of where military families live also has a negative impact on military spousal employment opportunities as active-duty spouses tend to live in locations that are saturated with other military spouses and this has a negative effect on spousal employment (Booth et al., 2000). Active-duty military spouses are predominantly young females with education, work experiences, and skills similar to those of their peers. Since the military moves families around so frequently, spouses acquire limited earning potential, less work experience, and interrupted work histories. Another complicating factor is that the military itself is an internal labor market and reserves most of its jobs for military personnel. Civilian jobs in the surrounding communities tend to be small in number and in low-paying service industries fueled with more supply than demand. Families who move frequently fall under the category of "migrant families" and these families relocate geographically based on employment demands of the highest wage earner in the family. Migrant families are similar to active-duty military families in that they move based on the employment demands of this highest earner, which is typically the service member. The difference between military and non-military families who move often is that non-military migrant families move based on shifts in the labor market and military families move by shifts in military training needs as well as shifting events in world politics. The combination of multiple geographic relocations, regular role shifts causing increased responsibilities in the family, decreased employment opportunities, and unstable employment histories cause many military spouses to become increasingly dependent (over time) financially on the service member. At the same time, these spouses are not able to develop the necessary experience, skills, and careers they would need to be independent and/or to become the primary wage earner should they or the family require this at any point in the future.

Military spouses of active-duty service members face unique challenges to securing and maintaining employment in the civilian labor market. Employers are hesitant to hire military spouses because they need to move every few years and they lose the long-term benefits of workers they trained and supported to be productive. In terms of a business model and a cost–benefit ratio, an employer's investment in a military spouse as a worker is a financial loss for a company, unless that work can be virtual and across state lines. In terms of the supply-and-demand theory of economics, the labor pool of available workers in and around military installations is large and saturated with applicants of similar age, education, and training/experience. These situational factors combine to make securing paid labor extremely difficult for military spouses. In one study conducted with employed spouses of military service members, the majority of them reported that being a military spouse negatively affected their work opportunities and cited frequent moves as the primary reason (Castaneda & Harrell, 2008). In addition to moves, spouses with children also reported that deployment-related absences of the service members contributed to work-related problems, as they assumed full responsibility for childcare and domestic work in the home during these separations. These spouses also expressed frustration over these issues even when the service members were not absent, reflecting a possible conflict between the conservative values and traditional gender roles present in many military families and a societal shift away from these in the civilian population. The perception that there is employer bias against hiring, training, and promoting military spouses was also mentioned by these spouses as having a negative effect on their work opportunities. In addition to these, occupational licensure and certification were also mentioned as factors that negatively impact employment situations and career trajectories especially with moves to different states that tend to have their own licensing requirements (Castaneda & Harrell, 2008).

In 2011, the DoD responded to the chronic levels of unemployment, underemployment, and documented wage gap between military and civilian spouses by expanding the Army Spouse Employment Partnership from its original inception in 2003 to include active-duty spouses from the other branches of the military (Navy, Marine Corps, and Air Force) seeking private-sector careers (Gonzalez et al., 2015). The Military Spouse Employment

Partnership reported having approximately 300 organization members committed to recruiting, hiring, promoting, and retaining military spouses. This program is one of four initiatives of the Spouse Education and Career Opportunities (SECO) program under the Assistant Secretary of Defense for Readiness and Force Management's Military Community and Family Policy Office. The continuing goals of the SECO program are to address unemployment and underemployment among military spouses, match education and experience to available employment positions, and to close the wage gap between military spouses and their civilian counterparts (Gonzalez et al., 2015). The components of service delivery for the SECO program include: My SECO, an online portal that provides virtual tools and resources to promote educational achievement and employment attainment; the Military OneSource SECO Career Call Center staffed by certified career counselors to provide services at no cost; and the My Career Advancement Account Scholarship that provides up to $4,000 of tuition assistance for licensure and educational benefits for spouses.

The Military Spouse Preference applies to spouses of active-duty military service members including full-time National Guard members who relocate to a new duty station. It provides hiring preference for active-duty military spouses who can submit PCS orders and gain increased points when applying for government jobs through USAjobs.gov, the government employment website, or other federal hiring agencies. This preference is not available to military spouses in the National Guard and Reserves who do not relocate as geographic mobility is believed to be the most significant concern by the government-sponsored program. In 2018, Executive Order 13832 called "Enhancing Noncompetitive Civil Service Appointments of Military Spouses" expanded the definition of military spouse to include spouses of medically disabled (retired or separated) service members, and spouses who are widows or widowers (not remarried) of a service member killed while performing active-duty military service. This policy was set to enhance support for military spouses, help retain service members, enhance military readiness, and decrease the burden of regulations that can inhibit the entry of military spouses into the workforce. The multiple and frequent relocations were listed in this policy as making it challenging for military spouses to maintain the "home front," comply with licensure and job requirements, and to obtain adequate childcare. Following the enactment of this policy, military spouses of veterans who have military-connected injuries and disability ratings with the V.A. are entitled to a 10-point bonus in their applications for federal employment opportunities. Further policy initiatives to address geographic relocations that negatively affect military spouses include unemployment compensation eligibility for military spouses across state lines and inter-state endorsement of professional licenses for military spouses. The inter-state professional licensure policy shift has been problematic for many spouses as not all states have adopted its use to date and spouses are advocating for federal licensing for military spouses at this time.

The lack of gainful employment available to many spouses of active-duty service members leaves them without significant opportunities for building both internal and external resources that could help to sustain them throughout the often-difficult life transitions associated with military family life. A lack of engagement with the labor force leaves these spouses in a void without that network of support that come from formal (workplace, compensation, benefits) and informal (relationships with co-workers, group activities, career mentoring) sources. The result of this situation for many spouses is that they are isolated from opportunities to build career and social networks to develop financial stability that would help them at the time as well as prepare them for their family's transition to civilian life after military service. These spouses do not gain access to the support that comes from a sense of belonging to a community outside of the nuclear family; such a community would care about their well-being and membership in it would likely encourage higher levels of resiliency for these spouses and their family system. Given the substantial burden faced by military families after prolonged wars and multiple deployments, access to targeted and effective programming informed by research on these topics is greatly needed at this time as there are more than one million current active duty military spouses and more than 15 million spouses of veterans in the United States (Borah & Fina, 2017).

Of these spouses, an estimated 1.1 million individuals provide informal care to veterans who served since September 11, 2001 and since many service members married young, many of these caregivers are spouses who are younger than in previous wars (Miller et al., 2015). According to a recent RAND report, post-9/11 veterans tend to be younger than veterans who served prior to 9/11, with 46% aged 18–30 years and 94% younger than 55 years (Ramchand et al., 2014). In response to the needs of caregivers, Public Law 111–163, the Caregivers and Veterans Omnibus Health Services Act of 2010, was passed to provide support, education, training, and assistance for caregivers of veterans. As 33% of caregivers of younger, post-9/11 veterans are spouses, they are adopting the role of caregiver at a younger age and it remains unclear whether programs needed during the initial adjustment to the role will be needed indefinitely if they spend time on caregiving instead of becoming employed in the labor force (Ramchand et al., 2014).

There is evidently more research needed to discover reasons and generate solutions for the high unemployment and underemployment rates of civilian spouses married to military service members. Although these spouses have time to develop career paths following the family's military service, the experience of chronic unemployment, underemployment, reduced wages, and/or employment that is mismatched with one's skills and education levels has lasting implications. More research with military spouses would help to understand their experiences and to determine long-term effects on health, wellness, and career paths of civilian spouses. Research has examined the effects of chronic unemployment on the veteran population repeatedly over time due to this significant risk factor and studies found that long-term unemployment had worse effects for veterans than their civilian counterparts (Tran, Canfield, & Chan, 2017). Similar research with military spouses would be highly beneficial in terms of public health policies directed at improving civilian spousal employment and in gaining a better understanding of the effects of spousal unemployment on individuals and families.

DoD programs designed to improve the employment situations for civilian spouses of active-duty service members could be evaluated for their effectiveness across several domains. The situations that could be included are as follows: finding and maintaining employment in one's chosen occupation; employment that does not match the appropriate level for the spouse's skills, training, and professional development; the spouse's health and mental health outcomes; the family's level of functioning; and the family's fiscal management of the economic gains of the increased family earnings. The results could factor in the job performance of the military service member to ascertain whether gains in civilian spousal employment have positive or negative associations in terms of role shifts due to spousal employment. Civilian spousal employment research would not only help to better understand military families, but it would also provide more detailed information about the links between family readiness, retention, military occupational performance, and caregiving roles filled in military families.

Single Parenting Demands and Deployments

Service members who are single parents are twice as likely to be female than male and more likely to be enlisted than officers with approximately 5% of active-duty and 9% of National Guard/Reserve members being single parents (DoD, 2013). Single-parent service members are required to identify a caregiver in cases of deployment and failure to be able to set up an alternative family care plan can result in being designated for "non-deployable" status or having alternate administrative actions to manage. In addition to the length of a deployment, the quality and intensity of risk that is perceived by the family or caregivers are contributing factors that influence the family's overall response as these characterize the level of threat to the system. There are external mediating factors that influence a family's response to stressful situations, including social supports outside of the family system such as the formal and informal support networks available to the military family that are protective in nature. Social networks are based on good will and friendships that develop throughout one's life and these social connections can create strong ties that share responsibility for members and collective competence from being part of a larger community. Formal support networks are those that are found in such places as schools, alumni associations, athletic memberships/health clubs, religious, and/or places or organizations of employment. They are the formal ties to all the communities outside of the family. Informal networks include friendships, support groups, neighbors, and people who work or visit other members of the community that families interact with on a regular basis.

Families Navigating Separation and Loss

Military spouses who remain at home during a service member's deployment face a number of challenges that encompass internal well-being and external factors that influence how the period of separation will be experienced. Spouses who have histories that include depression, trauma, or significant losses in their past, for example, will be at heightened risk during a military deployment from the temporary loss and the threat of permanent loss of the service member. These spouses will be at risk for depression during a deployment and would benefit from increased social support during this time to increase their overall capacity to manage the stressful situation. The meaning that is attached to the deployment by the spouse is significant as the spouse's perception of threat to the service member will be an influencing factor in the family's overall stability. In situations where the perception of danger does not match the reality of the deployment situation, increased communication could prove impactful for increasing family resiliency. In the event that the increased communication cannot be a comforting factor, such as if the deployment is dangerous or the service member reports concerns about such incidents involving chaotic situations, lack of unit cohesion, and/or problematic leadership, then the communication would not be comforting to the spouse and family and would reinforce the spouse's fears around safety. If the spouse fears for the safety of the service member on a deployment, there is greater likelihood that they will also fear for the survival of the family unit if the service member is killed in action or does not return home. Deployments that involve long periods of separation with an ever-present threat of death can remind spouses and family members of losses that were significant in the past and the associated feelings can easily return to complicate the family's well-being.

Socioeconomic factors such as financial strain, job stress, and number of dependents were found to all negatively impact spousal well-being due to the increased levels of responsibility that need to be assumed by the military spouse (Donoho et al., 2018). The higher degree of responsibility combined with the associated role changes in the family can lead to the spouse experiencing increased anxiety. The spouse's psychological well-being will impact the family's overall ability to cope adaptively to the stress at home during a deployment and decreased mental health functioning places the family at risk for maladaptation to emerge as a result. One study on the effects of deployment on military spouses identified some of the risk factors related to increased depression including education, employment, number of children, and military component are associated with the diagnosis of major depressive disorder (Donoho et al., 2018). Another study reported that inadequate support from the military was the most frequently reported response relating to spousal distress (Runge et al. 2014). The military lifestyle comes with challenges that involve geographically relocating often which causes disruptions in social networks, friendships, and sense of stability. As one spouse reported: "Not a single Army person called me to see how I was doing while my husband was in Afghanistan for 10 months and I was at home looking after our baby" (Runge, et al. 2014). This statement highlights the desire, and the need, for the military to accept the responsibility for the deployment and take action steps to reach out to spouses during deployments also known as "welfare checks" on a regular basis.

Research suggests that spouses that are able to prioritize family in a cohesive manner while communicating effectively have a decreased risk of distress (Sullivan et al., 2021). This is reflective of a spouse remaining present and engaged with their family members rather than closed off and distant. Essentially, the coping mechanisms that are uniquely developed by the spouse and family system while their partner is deployed is crucial for meeting the demands of being a military family. Some major themes of coping for military spouses were inclusive of taking on the responsibilities of their spouse, seeking an outlet for distraction, and having the hope to remain strong throughout the deployment phase (Marnocha, 2012). Being able to successfully take on the role of the deployed spouse while also successfully balancing their own, displayed the flexibility of military spouses' capability greatly. In one study, a spouse of a service member responded to a survey regarding the emotional process during the deployment phase and shared, "You're just stuck and you have to go with it. I could either let this break me down or I can let it make me stronger, and that's just what I did" (Marnocha, 2012). This sense of self-determination and hope to thrive amongst hardship and isolation is a mentality developed by military spouses to cope with new challenges in order to overcome the adverse stressors that present during deployment. Ultimately, military spouses "learned to effectively manage emotions and use their support systems to help them stay strong" as a source of resiliency (Marnocha, 2012). It was also found that social support, although a risk factor, can be recognized as a protective factor for resiliency within a military family. The contention that "decreased isolation and increased social support have been associated with lower stress" allows for spouses to act on the available resources provided to them through the military and their community in order to prevail against the challenges of deployment (Sullivan et al., 2021). By refraining from isolation and engaging in support groups, community activities, and spending time with friends and family, military spouses are able to create a new support system.

Military spouses who experience isolation and/or depression are at increased risk for reduced resiliency during stressful situations including relocations, trainings, deployments, and reintegration challenges in the couple's marital relationship. It is crucial for military spouses to become aware of their feelings and internal psychological experiences to be able to identify mental health challenges that may interfere with resiliency as soon as they arise. As depression and other forms of internal distress tend to impair communication patterns and limit the cognitive flexibility necessary for resiliency, early identification and treatment, and building social support systems are all key components for military family resiliency. Seeing as one of the largest themes for resiliency during deployment was access to adequate social support, a program engineered to specifically address spousal concerns, challenges, and needs during the deployment phase can be extremely helpful for developing productive and meaningful coping strategies. For instance, offering support groups and building support networks for military spouses would provide a sense of community and belonging during stressful times such as during the absence of their loved one. Military families who do not reside on a military base experience a scarcity of resources and are at risk for social isolation and barriers to accessing support networks that could enhance resiliency. By increasing social support and community connections, military spouses and other significant family members feel less isolated and are able to share the burden of their lived experience with other family members in their local non-military community. A challenge that may arise to military spouses seeking help from providers and the community is the impact of the stigma within the military that asking for help continues to be limited due to perceptions. It is estimated that roughly 20% of active-duty military spouses are reluctant to seek mental health treatment or support due to stigma, perceived weakness/failure, embarrassment, and fears that it would have a negative effect on the service member's career (Verdeli et al., 2011). Reshaping the military culture to encourage mental health treatment as a positive, prosocial, resilient response to stress would go a long way to improving spousal distress and improving the overall quality of life for many military families. A useful analogy is often one between mental health and physical health in that physical therapy for a broken bone or other physical injury works to help an individual repair what is hurting and to get back to optimal levels of performance in daily life. Mental health therapy is similar in that it helps an individual repair what is distressing (hurting) so they can get back increased levels of functioning in daily life, psychologically and behaviorally.

Affect Management Styles in Families

Families have many diverse ways and styles for communicating a range of experiences from reporting day-to-day happenings to sharing highly personal emotions, internal thoughts, and affective reactions to life events and to one another. This section explores some of these differences as well as some of the cultural attributes and contexts that contribute to the underlying patterns for communications. Some families are considered "highly expressive" and daily interactions are filled with heightened affective states and intense emotional reactions whereas other families are reserved in their interactions and rarely express affects or emotions. The topic of affect management is helpful in understanding how individuals both experience and process strong emotional states internally and how they communicate these states to family members and significant others in their lives. The internal experience of affect management is understood in terms of how an individual regulates their emotions and what happens when this ability is overwhelmed due to stress or other factors. The result of not being able to manage one's emotions is that the individual may become flooded with emotions and dysregulated in their internal world which in turn can influence their behaviors in their external world. In terms of family functioning, when individual family members are overwhelmed by stress, with regular dysregulated affective states present in the system, the predictability of family life is removed and the stability of the family is no longer experienced.

Affect management in family communication is a critical resiliency skill that makes collaborative problem solving possible when emotions are heightened in stressful situations. In addition to affect management, the related concepts of distress tolerance and mindfulness will be reviewed as therapeutic techniques for building communication resiliency skills to be able to manage strong affective states that arise in response to crises. The skills for managing strong negative emotions without acting on them are found in the techniques of dialectical behavior therapy that has developed over time and is currently generalized for its usefulness in therapeutic settings through an educational focus on mental health (Linehan & Wilks, 2015). The incorporation of the combined skills of affect management, distress tolerance, and mindfulness techniques are understood to be ways for building family resiliency to stress. These skills are present in the diverse ways in which families express feelings, manage stress overall, and develop unique communication styles that will be examined in this section as well.

The differences in communication styles found in families has a direct impact on family functioning and overall family resiliency. Open and honest communication is one of the measures of healthy relationship functioning in families and these interactional patterns can best be established during periods of relative stability in family life. Healthy communication patterns that are present or developed during stability in the home environment will serve as protective factors for resiliency in times of stress and crisis. Military families that are highly expressive by nature in times of stability yet unable to be open and honest during deployments are likely to experience different challenges than families who tend to operate on a daily basis at home with low levels of communication. Families are forced to adjust their communications during a deployment and develop new ways for communicating that are challenging in terms of the amount (quantity) of the communication as well as the style (quality) of the interactions during the separation period. The crisis of the deployment separation demands that all families adapt to the change and the ways in which they adapt has a significant impact on the functioning of the family system as well as how it will recover from the crisis.

Adults living with unresolved childhood trauma are at risk for experiencing traumatic stress reactions that may have been dormant, or coped with in maladaptive ways, for years to emerge if living with a partner who is experiencing active PTSD. Couples may become fearful and defensive of one another, rigid and inflexible, and engage in battles for dominance and control that erupt in attachment rage, often vacillating between approach and avoidance in the relationship (Basham, 2008). Military service members/veterans and their partners often do not understand these relationship dynamics or the devastating power that trauma has to challenge even the strongest attachment bonds. Military couples will often blame themselves or believe that they have failed in the relationship somehow and may easily fall into states of depression as a result. When this happens, military couples are at increased risk for new stressors to emerge from maladaptive coping behaviors including substance use, family conflict, and marital/couple infidelity. Military couples struggling with PTSD and unresolved childhood trauma can benefit greatly from psychoeducation around these relationship dynamics in a culturally sensitive manner that increases their understanding and family resiliency (Herzog, Whitworth, & Scott, 2020). The risk factors of combat stress and childhood trauma in military couples heighten the family's overall risk for maladaptation to the stressful situation of reintegration and need a thorough assessment and exploration of the couple's histories at the beginning of any treatment. In addition to direct communication through psychoeducation about the effects of trauma on military families in stress, clinicians need to educate their clients about the benefits of affect management and boundary setting in family relationships.

Affect management and boundary setting can mean different things to different people and is highly subjective to the individual or family. Due to the nature of the military culture, training, and lifestyle, the concept and term "affect management" may sound very similar to the process of suppressing or "cutting off" from one's feelings. Psychoeducation around affect management in military families needs to include making the clear distinction that managing one's affects does not mean suppressing one's feelings and family members can learn the skills for identifying feelings and tolerating those feelings. These skills are helpful in connection with unresolved childhood trauma and overwhelming affective emotional states for individuals experiencing traumatic stress in their relationships. Military families who are struggling with traumatic stress reactions also need to strengthen their interpersonal boundaries in order to establish the sense of safety needed for traumatic stress to heal and resolve in adaptive ways. The typical traumatic response in relationships is "approach and avoidance" with the approach to significant loving attachment bonds experienced as potentially life threatening. The reaction to this is avoidance which is reminiscent of the early childhood attachment reaction of being dismissive and detached, turning away from a significant attachment bond, and denying one's feelings of disappointment and frustration. Military service members are often very familiar with the process of detaching from one's feelings to be able to engage in military missions that would otherwise be impossible if one experienced the range of emotions during trainings and on the battlefield. During the reintegration following wartime deployments, this coping skill often continues, and military families in treatment need new coping skills to be able to replace these military detachment skills and behaviors.

Military Family Crises in Deployments

According to Hill's (1949) research, there are at least three variables at work to determine whether a given event becomes a crisis for a family: (1) The hardships of the situation or event itself; (2) The resources of the family, its role structure, flexibility, and previous history with crisis; and (3) The definition the family makes of the event; that is, whether family members treat the event as if it were or as if it were not a threat to their status, their goals, and objectives. There are several situations that define a crisis for a family such as an adolescent depression, substance abuse issue, or an unplanned pregnancy for a military youth. There are a few different types of family crises such as the crisis of Accession, which is the addition of an unprepared-for family member, such as in an adolescent pregnancy. If a family crisis emerges at the same time as a parental military deployment, it may be defined as a crisis when at other times of relative calm it may not rise to the same level of distress and have as great of an impact on family functioning. The event of a death in a family would be considered a crisis of Dismemberment and would lead to increased challenges should it happen during a deployment and could result in the family experiencing a third crisis called Demoralization. The crisis of Demoralization is defined by Hill (1949) as the potential loss of morale and family unity. In families who employ Open Ranks as their style of adapting to the loss of the service member, they will leave some of the service member's roles unfilled and there will not be significant changes to how the family functions daily as they wait out the return of the service member. Families who utilize Closed Ranks as their style of adaptation to the stressful situation of a deployment will not be likely to inform the military member about important family information and that person's roles and responsibilities in the family will be taken on by other family members. The crisis of Demoralization can occur when either of these styles of adapting to the role exit and loss of the service member fail to meet the demands needed for successful family coping that would be evidenced by stability in daily routines and levels of functioning.

In times of crisis, disruptive transitions, or prolonged stress, communication is more likely to break down at the very time when it is needed the most and clarity in the midst of open emotional expression results in collaborative problem-solving in families (Walsh,

2016). Families who do not manage their crises well will grow apart rather than coming together as a family unit and will struggle to solve their problems with communication skills that are underdeveloped or deteriorating as a result of the crisis situation. Families with minimal or no communication between family members lack clarity, open communication, affection, and empathy toward one another during a difficult time. These families will also tend to be challenged in their abilities to tolerate and cope with the many painful feelings that arise as a result of the family separation, loss, and all of the associated events going on within the family. Instead of talking to each other and listening to everyone's needs, some family members are likely to seek support outside the family and in terms of adolescent risk factors, these may be peer groups with negative influences in terms of alcohol abuse or substance use.

Families who interact with poor communication styles tend to talk less about emotions, have difficulty comforting each other, utilize greater avoidance strategies, and have few positive family interactions; this often leads to tension and fear to emerge as a result of not allowing for open emotional expression between family members (Walsh, 2016). Families who interact with effective communication styles in times of deployment separation and loss facilitate emotional regulation and foster emotional closeness among family members as open communication allows for emotional expression, intimacy, and positive interactions during stressful times such as the crisis of a deployment separation. Effective communication is the result of a variety of skills including clarity, which facilities effective family functioning and makes it easier to cope with the stressful situation through clear and consistent verbal and behavioral messages that lead to shared understandings. Shared understanding helps to clarify ambiguous information and truth seeking. Open emotional expression helps a family to share both painful and positive feelings (such as appreciation, affection, and sadness) when dealing with adversity and resilience is facilitated by the ability of members to express and tolerate a wide range of feelings from the negative to the positive. Collaborative problem solving is a skill in families that entails shared decision-making and helps in the practice of creative brainstorming together of problematic situations.

Although communication is one of the hallmarks of resiliency in family functioning, it is common in families who are experiencing stressful situations to have problematic communications with one another during these times. The topic of remaining open and honest in family communication is a key component in the ways in which resilient families operate as well as the ability to navigate times when communication paths shut down. Communicating openly to share information and relay emotions in an honest manner is a necessary component for family resiliency and a skillset that can be learned and/or enhanced within families. Families that are not able to communicate effectively are at very high risk for utilizing negative coping strategies and developing systemic adaptations that are unhealthy during stressful situations. A family system that is not resilient to stress is vulnerable to conflicts developing or worsening between individual family members as misperceptions take root and overall family functioning suffers as a result. Misperceptions develop in the absence of open communication and the sharing of information is vital to correct misperceptions and their related behaviors.

The many and varied ways in which diverse families manage stress need to consider the dynamic interplay between adaptations that either build or deplete a family's overall resiliency. The concepts of family adaptation to stress and their impact on resiliency is generalizable to all families, including civilians who are not in military families. Individual and family risk factors need to be identified that impede resiliency and specifically those that concern perceptions around trust and safety in relationships can be shifted into more positive perceptions to improve resiliency. According to Walsh (2016), families that experience breakdowns in communication processes also experience related negative effects. Breakdown of clarity in family communication leads to ambiguous information across the family system that has not been clarified as there is no consistent messaging between members that would clarify such ambiguity in factual information as well as in individual perceptions of the problem and their roles such that some may blame themselves or other family members based on this ambiguous information. Breakdown of open emotional expression leads to a lack of sharing of the range of emotions from painful feelings to positive feelings and families need such expression to maintain the sense of connectedness and cohesion to be effective as a system (Walsh, 2016). Families that are able to tolerate differences between individual members are able to use the coping skill of mutual empathy to stay connected throughout situations of increased stress and adversity. Open emotional expression also involves taking responsibility for one's own feelings and behavior, avoiding blaming other family members for situations, and affirming the family's strengths while building on its potential to overcome challenges. Positive and healthy adaptation in the face of adversity over time requires enhanced psychobiological regulation of stress as well as optimal affect regulation skills so the individual does not become overwhelmed by reactions to stressful situations.

Collaborative problem solving relies on family members who practice open emotional sharing, effective communication skills, and collaborative goal setting in families. Problem solving also relies on adaptability and flexibility when needed to deal with family crises, communication about difficult issues, adjustment to shifts in family dynamics, and consensus of the identification of the problem and the family's perception of it. Collaborative problem solving requires awareness of the problem, a shared definition of the crisis, agreement on a solution, and adaptive coping strategies to improve family communications following the resolution of the crisis. A breakdown in collaborative problem solving leads to limited intra-family resourcefulness, no shared decision-making, few attempts to repair conflicts, being reactive in times of situational crises, and little preparation for future challenges (Walsh, 2016). Crisis in change of status and quality of the relationships between children and parents may be equally impacted as well during a deployment separation (Hill, 1949). A family crisis with negative changes in the quality of familial relationships has the potential to lead to attachment anxiety characterized by avoidance in significant relationships as a resulting maladaptive coping response. Every family member has socially prescribed roles that they play in the family's life up until those roles no longer meet the demands of a situation such as the crisis of a deployment separation. The individual functions as a member of the family largely in terms of the expectations other members place upon him or her and the family succeeds, or fails at adaptation to the stressful situation, based upon each member's role performance. The crisis (deployment) causes change within these role patterns especially when members are not living up to the expectations of other family members. The key ingredients of successful adaptation to deployment stress in military families require several conditions to be present within the family. These include the recognition of interdependence of all members upon one another; the satisfaction of playing one's roles in the family, whatever they are; the sharing of home management duties among all members; the flexibility of the family when facing new situations; the adequacy of intra-family communication; and opportunities for growth and development in the family environment. Previous experience with crises offers excellent clues both as to the outcome of the family in the new crisis as well as to the pattern of adjustment the family will follow (Hill, 1949).

Interpersonal Violence in Military Families

Military families are at increased risk for heightened stress levels due to the many demands of the military lifestyle, frequent trainings, and deployment cycles with risk involved. Veteran status has been associated with up to three times the rate of intimate partner violence than civilians and veterans are more likely than civilians to cause significant injury as a result (Taft et al., 2016; Marshall et al., 2005). Risk factors for intimate partner violence include depression, anger, social isolation, marital conflict/instability, and a lack of broader social connections, many of which are seen in reactions to deployment stress in military families. In one study, approximately 35,000 U.S. Air Force active-duty members and 24,000 civilian spouses in 82 military installations across the United States, Europe, and Asia completed the 2006 Community Assessment, an anonymous online survey assessing interpersonal violence (IPV) together with risk and protective factors (Smith et al., 2014). This study proposed an ecological model for IPV prevention that focuses on the individual, couple, and community levels for resources and support networks available there.

Community support, measured by the perceptions of support available in the community, as well as the level of community cohesion, serves to be a protective factor in reducing IPV in families. Communities with high rates of poverty and neighborhood disorder (perceived levels of neighborhood problems) were associated with higher levels of IPV. The authors reported that financial stress was associated with IPV perpetration and contributing risk factors included: increased depressive symptoms, decreased personal coping abilities, decreased physical well-being, and decreased relationship satisfaction. Community support was a protective factor against IPV, as it improved individual functioning. Spouses and partners who received support in primary healthcare were less likely to experience IPV, a correlation mediated by relationship satisfaction, thought to be linked to public awareness of the violence preventing it. Another study on the effects of community support on IPV for civilian couples of Hispanic/Latino backgrounds found specific variables that were risk factors along gender lines (Cunradi, 2009). The study found that for men, neighborhood disorder was associated with IPV perpetration and victimization; and for women, neighborhood disorder and the risk factor of their own alcohol abuse were both associated with IPV victimization but not IPV perpetration. These studies confirm previous literature linking community support and community cohesion to improved individual and couple functioning, reduced levels of IPV, and overall family well-being with reduced child maltreatment as a result. Given that studies have shown that alcohol and substance abuse are overrepresented among IPV perpetrators (two thirds of men in batterer intervention programs and approximately half of the women arrested for domestic violence), this variable is a serious risk factor to consider in building family safety, stability, and resiliency (Stover, Easton, & McMahon, 2013).

The rates of domestic violence in the military are consistently higher than in the civilian population and a Department of Defense program called Military OneSource provides information, resources, and referrals to all military families who choose to use it voluntarily. According to this program, the Department of Defense defines domestic abuse as a pattern of behavior that results in several different situations. IPV includes physical, sexual, emotional, and psychological abuse, which may include excessive jealousy, personal insults, verbal harassment, as well as threatening language suggesting the use (or future use) of physical abuse. IPV includes economic control of one partner by the other; one partner may control how the other spends money, intentionally accumulating credit card debt in the other person's name or refusing to share the decision-making on household finances. IPV interferes with one's personal freedom, which includes tracking the victim through electronic devices, apps or social media, or forbidding the victim to leave the home. IPV includes spousal neglect, in which one spouse or partner fails to provide the necessary care or assistance to the other spouse or partner in the event they are physically, emotionally, or culturally incapable of self-care. The use, attempted use, or threatened use of physical force is IPV and an offense under the Uniform Code of Military Justice, as well as state and federal laws. The Department of Defense defines an intimate partner as a current or former spouse; a person with whom the alleged abuser shares a child in common; a current or former intimate partner with whom the alleged abuser shares or had shared a home together; and any person who is (or has been) in a social relationship of a romantic nature.

The DoD created the Family Advocacy Program (FAP) to address issues of military family violence including child abuse and neglect. The FAP responds to reports of family violence and offers referrals to counseling as well as safety planning for victims involved in reported cases. There are two ways for reporting incidents of domestic violence in active-duty military families: restricted and unrestricted reporting. Restricted reporting is confidential and if a service member is the alleged perpetrator of family violence, neither they, nor their command, nor law enforcement are notified of the report. Restricted reporting is only available to adult victims who receive their medical care from a military treatment facility to assist them with safety planning, clinical crisis counseling, and minor medical treatment. This option is not available if there is a serious injury or the possibility of serious injury to anyone involved and is not available for situations of child abuse or neglect. In an unrestricted report, the military command and legal authorities receive notification of the report, which can increase the risk level for family members depending on how the situation unfolds. If the report leads to the service member's discharge from the military, the family will be at increased risk for losing military benefits such as base housing, schooling, income, and financial security.

Interpersonal family violence that is based on issues of power and control places military families at risk due to a combination of contextual factors surrounding the nature of the military organization. The military is an organization with a hierarchical structure of power and control for the purpose of the use of force as a weapon. Although career promotions entail multiple changes in roles, duties, and expectations in the military organizational structure, role confusion and role ambiguity in the family are likely to be threatening to the stability of the military family structure. Military families living amidst this cultural context, as well as families with prior military service, may have difficulty and not be able to tolerate levels of flexibility in role structures in the family. Veterans who hold traditional gender stereotypes may experience more discomfort with the presence of role ambiguity and this could lead to conflicts within the family until such confusion is resolved. In terms of family life transitions, deployments often serve as catalysts that force family members into positions of independence and task-centered competency. It is important to assess whether the at-home family members wanted role changes or assumed certain roles unwanted. An example of this might be a spouse or older adolescent child who takes on responsibilities and roles before they are emotionally prepared for them and struggles to succeed in fulfilling these new roles and the tasks involved. When these tasks involve caregiving responsibilities for younger children in the home, such situations may be detrimental to the caregiving process if the older sibling is not able to perform this role for the family, which will result in new problems or crises to emerge. The older sibling may take on responsibilities that he or she is unprepared to do, and this can place the younger children at risk for neglect, maltreatment, or inconsistent caregiving.

Given the alarmingly high incidence of domestic violence among military families, this problem requires more research and study into the reasons behind these prevalence rates.

Many theories link the presence of chronic and untreated posttraumatic stress from combat to certain triggers in one's environment or relationship that cause episodic rage and place the perpetrator of the violence at borderline levels of functioning during these episodes. Marital discord can certainly cause a reaction that is akin to the "escalation of force" discussed previously that is a normative part of military training for some service members. Marital conflict can also be a trigger for a traumatic rage reaction and trauma reactions can easily lead to dissociative episodes where one is out of control of their own behaviors. Domestic violence often occurs in the midst of a pattern of automatic responses to perceived abandonment and associated feelings of jealousy and rage. The connection to a patterned response of anger may be indicative of a depression fueled by frustration and shattered expectations following military deployments.

If the role confusion and unspoken feelings around role competency lead to confusion and conflict, this speaks to the need to incorporate these discussions into family life and/or therapeutic treatments. The skill of communication among family members needs to be taught, encouraged, and practiced on a daily basis in order for it to become habitual and second nature in family life. In addition to increasing the quantity of the communications in a family, the quality of the communication should be effective as well, so that intentions and motivations are a regular part of family interactions. Trauma that is untreated and becomes chronic can often lead many individuals to experience great difficulty holding onto the two opposing views of positive and negative perceptions of other people simultaneously. The psychological process of "splitting" the motivations and behaviors of others into "good or bad" often occurs internally within a traumatized person as a means for establishing safety. Trust in other people and the world is one of the key areas of internal life affected by trauma with shifts and distortions in cognitions. Traumatized individuals often benefit from guidance in the form of therapeutic treatment or education for awareness around this pattern of responding that may be causing conflicts in social and intimate partner relationships.

A pattern of pervasive mistrust in others often accompanies insecure attachment patterns, and deep-seated abandonment fears from early childhood can lead to jealousy, rage, and a desire to control one's partner. Domestic violence advocates use a visual depiction to describe topics of power and control in a wheel that attributes many of these processes to traditional gender-based roles in family systems. The power and control wheel illustrates how perceived threats are rooted in traditional gender-based stereotypes that dictate specific behaviors and roles in the family. The presence of insecure attachment patterns in military couples can cause great anxiety about family roles, particularly role shifts toward independence and autonomy, and place such families at increased risk for violence. The military culture and lifestyle demands role shifts of periodic independence for spouses, yet these spouses are identified and referred to as being in the role of "dependent" on the service member and military at all times. When roles do not shift back following a deployment, some military couples experience role conflicts as a result, and this can lead to negative effects on relationship functioning, marital satisfaction, military family life and family well-being if not negotiated and resolved.

Following military deployment to a war zone, especially for individuals experiencing problems such as chronic traumatic stress, there is an increased risk for IPV, demonstrated in research with combat veterans diagnosed with PTSD who experienced a series of cognitive misperceptions following deployment when they had returned home to their partners and families (Taft et al., 2016). These veterans had developed vigilance to threats in a war zone that led them to enter into survival mode while on deployment that was inappropriate when they were at home and not in the war zone. The service members had a tendency to perceive unrealistic threats, exhibited hostile appraisal of events, overvalued an aggressive response to threats; and exhibited a lower threshold for responding to the threat. Complicating factors often found in IPV include depression, alcohol use problems; traumatic brain injury; power conflicts; trust issues; and self-esteem problems. Significant coping strategies were included in the treatment such as psychoeducation around anger-related thinking; realistic appraisals of threat and others' intentions; stress management; problem-focused versus emotion-focused coping strategies; and relaxation training for anger management.

The "Strength at Home" program is a manualized, psychoeducational group model designed for veterans and military couples experiencing relationship difficulties who are at risk of engaging in a pattern of physical IPV or coercive, controlling behavior. It is a brief trauma-informed dyadic group intervention to prevent IPV in returning male service members/veterans and their intimate female partners informed by a cognitive–behavioral social information processing model (Taft et al., 2016). At the core of this social information processing model is the concept that trauma shapes how we interpret and otherwise process information gathered from our social environment. Trauma exposure can produce biases and deficits in social information processing within couples that increase risk of family violence. The study found that service members/veterans and their female partners engaged in relatively lower frequency of physical IPV than in an alternative program, indicating that this educational program could be helpful in preventing physical violence in relationships to emerge. The program is currently offered at V.A. Medical Centers and on certain military bases, in addition to medical settings that serve military couples, and in family support groups during and following deployments. The program's results indicate that while supportive interventions may be helpful for military couples, trauma-informed cognitive and behavioral change strategies are more effective in preventing the development of IPV over time (Taft et al., 2016).

Family Adjustment and Adaptation to Stress Model (Case Example)

Jason was six years old when his father left Fort Liberty, North Carolina, for a six-month deployment to a location that was undisclosed to his family for security reasons. Jason, his baby brother, and mother knew that his father was an Army Ranger who went on missions often and sometimes with short notice. He would always come back full of excitement and proud of the adventures he had just had and the work he was doing in the U.S. Army. Jason's view of his father was that he would always "light up a room" whenever he entered it and his excitement and zest for life was felt from the moment his father woke him up in the morning to the second his head hit the pillow at night. His father had no trouble sleeping as he worked hard and often for long hours and seemed to have more energy than most other dads he met; he talked openly about his values and how they helped him make choices in life; and when needed, talked about his troubles with his family and his Army buddies as he had deep and lasting relationships with the people who were closest to him. SSG Tolland told Jason that he would be the "man of the house" whenever he left for military trainings or deployments and that he had great confidence that Jason would live up to his expectations in helping his mother out with the baby and around the house with chores while he was gone. Jason had just started First Grade when he left for the deployment and his father told him that he expected that Jason would be reading books by the time he returned in the spring.

When Jason's father returned from his deployment, Jason noticed a difference in him that he had never seen previously as his father would easily become distracted and appear to be "lost in his thoughts." His father withdrew from time to time from family discussions that they had typically had around the dinner table and these times were unpredictable to Jason. Jason and his dad often threw a baseball in their backyard or at the park on base, usually initiated by his father, but happily agreed to by Jason who loved spending time with him. Jason waited for his father to ask him to play but when it didn't happen, Jason would initiate and say he wanted to throw the ball around with him. His father would usually agree and say "sure kid" but the way that he said it was different than he used to say it. His voice lacked the enthusiasm it once had and when they played catch, his dad seemed less interested and engaged than he had been in the past. It was as if his dad had changed somehow but Jason couldn't put into words how he had changed; he was confused and unsure about what was going on. He would often have to repeat "dad" several times and louder each time before he would get his father's attention. His father didn't go back to waking Jason up in the morning and said that since he showed that he had been able to do it himself during the deployment with an alarm clock, he didn't need him to do this task anymore. He patted Jason firmer than he used to on the back, and said that he was proud of how "grown up" Jason had become that he no longer needed him so much. Since he craved his father's attention so much more than he had in the past, Jason never mentioned to his father that when he "patted" him on his back, sometimes it hurt because it was firmer than it had ever been before the deployment. He never said anything about this to anyone because he imagined this was the way that "grown up" sons were supposed to act and how they were shown affection by their fathers. Jason felt both sadness and confusion about these changes in roles and tasks because in his mind he was doing what he needed to do to get by without his father only until he returned and not because he had "grown up" in his absence. Jason wanted his dad to go back to the way that he was before he left and wanted their relationship to go back to what it was as well. Jason's dad had been fully engaged in his life and relationships and now the only way that Jason could describe him was "gone but not gone."

Although his dad was back home and back in his daily family life, he was distant and emotionally unavailable, and was keeping a very definite boundary up between his family and wherever it was that he went when he got lost in his thoughts. When they used to play catch together or laugh at family inside jokes, his dad would lock eyes with Jason, really look at him and see him, in a way that no one else ever did. They were in sync with one another at those times and the eye contact they held when they laughed and played together gave Jason the feeling that everything was going to be okay even when he had bad days at school. Jason couldn't make sense out of the changes in his relationship with his dad and when he tried asking his mother to explain what was going on, she denied that it was as serious as Jason was saying it was and told him "not to worry" and that his dad just needed "time to get over the deployment." Jason didn't know what that meant and when she told him not to worry, Jason realized that he was, in fact, very worried because he didn't understand what was going on in his family. He was insecure about his relationship with his father and his mother was acting as if nothing had changed and said she was "just happy to have him home alive and well." Jason needed an explanation himself for the changes and the conclusion he reached was one that was formulated by a six-year-old child on his own without adult input or clarification to assist him in this process. Having such limited information about relationships and in the absence of a clear explanation, Jason went over the four things he did know that concretely had happened in his family:

1. *His father had said that he expected him to be reading by the time he got back home;*
2. *Jason had had difficulty learning how to read and was behind his peers academically;*

3. *Jason had spent extra time making sure he set his alarm clock every night and woke up on his own every morning to fill the role that his father had done for him previously;*
4. *Jason's mother was not worried about his father so their marital relationship had not changed following his dad's return home.*

Based on these four facts, Jason came to the following conclusion to explain the changes in his relationship with his father: Jason's dad had told him that he expected him to be reading when he returned home and was disappointed in him for this so didn't want to play catch with him anymore because he thought Jason should be doing more homework; Jason also came to the conclusion that his dad was sad that Jason had grown up while he was gone so he pulled away from him because Jason didn't need him anymore and he no longer had to be in the role of "father" if Jason didn't need him for previous tasks in that role.

These conclusions formed Jason's perception of the situation that his father's behavior was because Jason had "grown up" and the changes were based in this change in their relationship, since his mother denied that she was worried about anything, and Jason blamed himself for the loss of his previous relationship with his father. Jason's perception of having caused his father to withdraw from him led Jason to become driven to excel academically, but not socially, and to become overly dependent on his father in an attempt to bring back their previous relationship that had become lost and filled with confusion around the meaning to a child of "growing up."

6 Trauma, Attachment, and Treatment Interventions

Military Families and Deployment Experiences

Many children experience shifts in their roles in the family during a parental deployment as well as several shifts and changes in the roles assumed by the non-deployed spouse. The developmental, emotional, and cognitive capabilities to understand a parent's deployment normatively increases with age in childhood and older youth are often placed in caregiver roles to younger siblings in the home. Adolescents from military families have reported high rates of hopelessness, sadness, depression, and suicidal ideation in the midst of family disruptions and reported to be at higher risk for substance use during or following a parental deployment (Acion et al., 2013). In addition to this, another study reported an increased rate of psychiatric hospitalization among military children between the ages of 9 to 17 years and reported that one of the significant stressors was a cumulative duration of time that the family had experienced parental deployments (Millegan et al., 2013).

Military spouses, family members, and significant others/partners who remain at home, without increased social support networks, and with histories or previous vulnerabilities toward anxiety or depression are at increased risk for emotional challenges during the deployment separation. If the parent at home experiences mental health challenges during these times, this may also impair the attachment bond between that caregiver and any children in the home. Children may feel less protected, safe, and stable if their primary caregiver experiences mental health challenges and decreased levels of functioning in the family as a result. In the absence of a strong support system to assist at-home caregivers who are vulnerable to mental health challenges through deployment phases, children are likely to experience emotional challenges themselves, often with accompanying maladaptive coping behaviors. Significant increased communication between families with video capabilities has occurred in recent years with the increased use of cell phones on deployments for service members. This ability for families to be in constant communication sometimes leads to increases in family stress levels as spouses and children become more aware of the challenges that their loved ones experience on deployment and service members see the emotional effects of the separation on their family at home. Deployments often cause military youth to experience anxiety and fears for the military parent's safety and the additional risk factor of decreased mental health functioning of the primary caregiver at home with disruptions in their attachment bond can easily lead to negative mental health outcomes for them. Military youth have reported higher rates of hospital visits, mental health issues, behavioral problems, and academic problems than non-military youth, with the longer the duration of the deployment, the higher the level of acuity of the problems experienced (Chandra et al., 2010).

Military couples often tend to avoid discussing issues that cause them anxiety while the service member is on a deployment such as financial difficulties, children's issues, family

DOI: 10.4324/9781003438229-9

problems, home management problems, sharing of painful feelings (including fears and anxieties surrounding the ever-present threat of death), traumatic events, morality, politics, and specifics of the deployment situation due to operational security. Couples who avoid talking about their feelings or certain topics during a deployment, however, place these issues at risk for becoming more difficult to bring up to discuss later when the deployment is over. Family life characterized by parental collusion of avoidance around conflictual issues and difficult feelings role models this behavior for children in the home who then are not able to develop healthy and adaptive communication patterns as they grow up. The at-home military spouse assumes the role of single parent during a deployment and takes on all the responsibilities for the management of the family. In doing so, the military spouse typically employs autonomous decision-making for the family, which is often difficult to give up when the deployment ends. Due to this probability, military couples may benefit from a division of responsibilities and mutually decide which decisions would involve the service member through shared information and collective problem-solving of family issues.

Military Sexual Assault

According to the Department of Defense, more than 5,200 service members reported a sexual assault in 2017 for an incident that occurred during their military service, an increase of about 10% from the previous year. According to recent estimates, most sexual assault victims do not seek immediate medical care, and studies have suggested that at least five out of every six sexual assaults are never reported to authorities. Sexual assault includes the following incidents: being physically forced into participation; unable to give consent; pressured with threats of consequences or promises of rewards; threatening, offensive remarks about a person's body or sexual activities; threatening and unwelcome sexual advances; unwanted touching or grabbing a person; oral sex, anal sex, sexual penetration with an object and/or sexual intercourse. Military sexual assault is an interpersonal trauma that may be repetitively ongoing over time and the victim may not have social support or assistance at the time. There are typically significant barriers to disclosing military sexual assault including stigma and the meaning that the military may attribute to the incident such as dismissiveness or blaming the victim. Sexual assault within the military culture and rank structure places additional barriers to reporting the assault due to multiple levels of power differentials present. In addition to this, the perpetrator of the assault may have friends in the military who collude with the incident through silence and secrets attributed to the military value of loyalty to peers in service. Mental health diagnoses associated with this sexual assault and trauma include PTSD, depression, increased suicidal behaviors, anxiety disorders; substance use disorders; eating disorders; dissociative disorders; and self-harming behaviors. Physical health conditions are also associated with headaches, gastrointestinal difficulties, chronic pain, chronic fatigue, and sexual dysfunction.

Military sexual assault/trauma often leads to self-blame, anger or aggression, and self-harming behaviors that develop amidst the multiple devastating consequences that follow such attacks. Self-blame can emerge in an attempt to make sense out of the event and to manage one's feelings that include a loss of control. Anger or aggression may emerge to offer the victim a sense of agency over one's life, isolate themselves for protection, and create emotional distance between them and potentially harmful people. Self-harm may serve to give some victims a controllable pain and to distract oneself from trauma-related thoughts or memories of the event. Although responses that emerge following sexual assault may offer temporary relief, these can prove maladaptive over time as self-blame can turn to feelings of depression, a poor self image, and poor choices; anger can decrease positive attachments and intimacy in relationships and lead to social isolation and difficulties in social settings; and self-harm can lead to feelings of shame and lost opportunities to learn to cope in ways that would otherwise foster positive adaptation and increased levels of confidence.

According to a recent report, nearly half of all the claims denied for PTSD related to military sexual assault/trauma were not properly processed (Sripada et al., 2018). Military sexual trauma includes sexual assault and/or sexual harassment that is threatening in nature and creates a hostile work environment; it can occur on or off base, while on or off duty and survivors on active duty are entitled to receive services at any V.A. Medical Center facility. Staff from the V.A. Benefits Administration (VBA) reported that the department had incorrectly processed approximately 1,300 of the 2,700 MST-related claims during the previous three years (49%). The reasons stated by the report for incorrectly processing MST reports included administrative or staff errors such as not requesting a medical examination or opinion despite sufficient evidence for one (28% of cases). In addition to this, staff did not request private medical treatment records or make required phone calls to the veterans. Staff also did not use the required language in letters sent to veterans to determine whether the veteran reported the event during military service, and often failed to obtain copies of those reports. V.B.A. staff also denied claims based on contradictory or insufficient medical opinions.

Invisible Wounds of War

Some of the more common injuries from military service include hidden or invisible wounds that are not visible yet greatly interfere with daily functioning and family life for those who sustain them. Traumatic brain injuries often co-occur and overlap with symptoms of posttraumatic stress when a service member sustains a head injury due to an incident that results in some degree of concussion. Many service-connected injuries from explosive devices resulted in concussions that are also known as traumatic brain injuries (TBIs), often with resulting PTSD from the incident, and other physical disabilities that negatively impact health, quality of life issues, and daily functioning. In situations where veterans sustained significant TBI with poly-trauma from military service, many families reported financial strain following the injury, with a depletion of assets and an accumulation of debt, and almost half of these spouses were forced to leave the labor force due to increased caregiving responsibilities at home (Van Houtven et al., 2013).

Traumatic brain injuries can range from mild to severe, cause long-term suffering, and chronic pain. Concussions that are defined as mild (TBI) represented the majority of cases in the post-9/11 wars according to the U.S. Department of Defense (2018). These concussions are traumatically induced disruptions of brain function that often results in loss of consciousness less than 30 minutes or an alteration of consciousness manifested by an incomplete memory of the event or being dazed and confused. Research is emerging on the impact of Low-Level Blast (LLB) exposure on brain health and functional abilities. Low-Level Blasts are blasts generated from firing heavy weapon systems or explosives in combat or training environments. While LLB exposure does not typically result in mild traumatic brain injury or concussion, service members and veterans in high-risk military occupations (such as combat arms units) have reported symptoms that include: concentration problems, chronic irritability, memory problems, reduced cognitive processing speed, decreased eye-hand coordination, hearing loss, headaches, and tinnitus in addition to specific behavioral changes. A moderate TBI consists of a loss of consciousness for more than 30 minutes, but less than 24 hours, and a confused or disoriented state that lasts more than 24 hours, and memory loss lasting greater than 24 hours but less than seven days. A severe TBI has a loss of consciousness for more than 24 hours; a confused or disoriented state that lasts more than 24 hours; and memory loss for more than seven days or more. The overwhelming majority of cases of mild TBIs were experienced in the Army at more than 225,000 reported cases between the years 2000–2017, followed by the Marine Corps at approximately 54,000; and the Navy and Air Force at approximately 52,000 for each branch of service (U.S. Department of Defense, 2018).

Some of the common symptoms following concussions include: headache, confusion, light-headedness, dizziness, nausea/vomiting, blurred vision, sensitivity to light, tired eyes, sensitivity to or loss of smell, tinnitus (ringing in the ears), fatigue/lethargy, changes in sleep patterns, trouble with memory, concentration, attention, and/or thinking, behavioral/mood changes such as depression, anxiety, irritability, and related issues. Persistent post-concussive symptoms (PPCS) occur when the symptoms of a mild traumatic brain injury last longer than is expected after the injury and often include headaches, sensitivity to light and sounds, dizziness, and problems with concentration and memory. The overlapping symptoms shared between TBI and PTSD make it difficult to separate the two conditions yet there are ones that are specific to both and are seen in Figure 6.1. The re-experiencing symptoms of re-living the images from the trauma, as well as feelings of guilt that may accompany PTSD, are not always present in the post-concussive sequelae of symptoms following a traumatic brain injury. The headaches, sensitivity to light, dizziness, and memory deficits that occur in concussions do not always co-occur with PTSD symptoms. The recovery from mild TBIs generally occurs within days, weeks, or months following the injury. At one week following a concussion, 90% of injured persons continue to report symptoms, whereas one month following the injury approximately 50% have fully recovered. At three months following the injury, approximately 66% have recovered. At 6–12 months post-concussion there are approximately 10% of injured who report symptoms and those who remain symptomatic at 12 months and longer are likely to have co-occurring complications.

Symptoms such as long-term problems with executive functioning, memory, and attention can interfere with family relationships and impair parenting largely due to chronic pain and difficulties with executive functioning. Pain management has led prescribers to multiple prescriptions of medications to alleviate distressing levels of pain that can lead to dependency and limit what may already be reduced involvement in family activities. Many of the overlapping symptoms with TBIs and traumatic stress include insomnia, interrupted sleep patterns due to the heightened stress response system, and changes in mood including depression, anxiety, irritability, and angry outbursts, all of which impair relationship

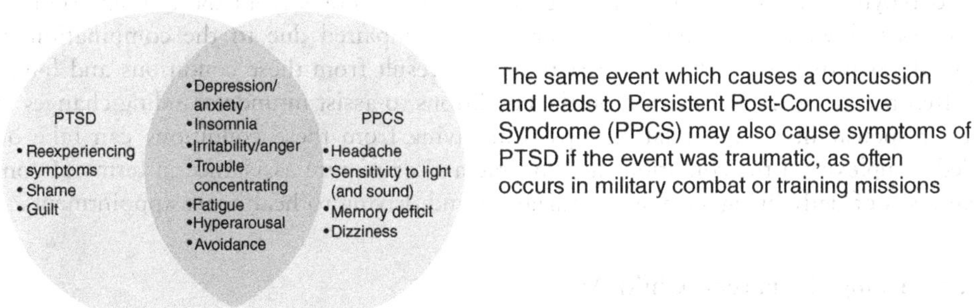

Figure 6.1 Overlap of PTSD and PPCS symptoms

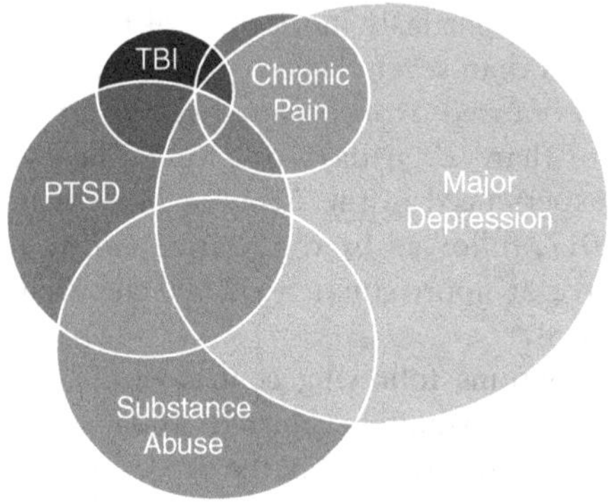

Figure 6.2 Co-occurring mental health concerns

functioning as a result. The reaction to the situation of being in combat, when one needs constant vigilance and physiological arousal for survival, does not easily turn off when a service member returns home following a deployment. Although service members have the opportunity to sleep through the night in the safety and security of being home with family, physiological reactions are not easy to shift, and can lead to unhealthy behaviors that all combine to create added stress in the family system.

Posttraumatic stress and mild traumatic brain injuries often stem from the same incidents in military service and tend to occur in tandem. Concussions from war-related situations are usually traumatic and include significant blasts from combat situations. The symptoms of PTSD include anxiety, avoidance, and social withdrawal that lead to reduced levels of functioning, difficulties in relationships, irritability, frustration expressing feelings, problems with trust, and difficulties with focus and concentration. Traumatic brain injuries are among the most prevalent injuries of the wars in Iraq and Afghanistan. TBIs among veterans from Iraq and Afghanistan vary between 9–28% during military service; however, many experienced at least one prior to their military service, complicating the healthcare trajectory for these veterans (Reger, Brenner, & du Pont, 2022). Many TBI symptoms occur in combination with PTSD symptoms due to the traumatic nature of sustaining a brain injury and behaviors such as avoidance, isolating, irritability, depression, aggression, and agitation are often difficult to tease apart (see Figure 6.2). Veterans with TBI can also experience physical and cognitive deficits, migraine headaches, tinnitus, poor balance, speech impairments, visual deficits, sleep disruptions, and impairments in short-term memory and executive functioning.

The invisible wounds of war have long-term implications for family functioning in the post deployment phase of family reintegration and symptoms from these often continue for years following returning home. Parenting is impaired due to the combination of physical, cognitive, and behavioral reactions that result from these conditions and families often need to gain information on the conditions to assist in understanding changes in roles, responsibilities, and relationships. Caregiving from these conditions can take on added complexity if the conditions are chronic and/or require assistance in terms of concrete tasks of daily living such as organization and driving to healthcare appointments.

Strengthening the Parent–Child Attachment

Children live in the context of their family and depend on their caregivers for their survival. In situations where these caregivers are physically, emotionally, or cognitively unavailable, they can easily become frightened and confused. Children constantly internalizing the messages they receive from adults in their lives as to how to handle stressful situations and without explanations for injuries, may become challenged in terms of adapting to the situation. Adults who are able to respond with resiliency and positive coping skills often have children who have learned healthy responses in times of crisis or increased stress and are able to respond with adaptive resiliency skills. Communication in resilient families is one of the key components to adaptive resiliency in times of stress and assisted by secure attachment patterns among family members. Parents and older children in resilient families are able to step outside themselves, monitor the situation, and disengage from negative interactions. Resilient families willingly disengage from negative interactions with one another because such negativity is viewed as more problematic than any one person's behavior, feelings, or reactions. Families that operate from a secure attachment base view one another as a respite, a comforting relief, and a solution to life's challenges and problems. Resilient families offer individual members a safe haven and protection when storms arise to challenge even the most resilient individuals. Family members give one another clear signals about what they need that facilitate those needs being met. There is trust that self-disclosures will be met with empathic responses that has been built up over time and confirmed in a repetitive fashion each time that it occurs again. The idea of the storm being actively present in family life would signal danger to a resilient family and the storm would be identified as the problem to be solved.

The storm would be considered threatening to the very fabric and infrastructure of that family as a secure, reliable, and effective operating system. In terms of behavior, resilient families do not withdraw from one another in times of stress nor communicate with hostility or aggression, as both of these would be perceived as threats to the survival of the system. In times of crisis or distress, if one family member exhibits emotions that appear out of control, this will represent a threat to the entire system, and resilient families will respond to help that person to become more in control of dangerous affective states. The previously developed secure attachment provides a protective internal layer of resiliency that allows the individual who is experiencing overwhelming feelings (such as rage or terror) to accept comfort and soothing from family members. The secure attachment bonds in resilient families are the keys that help individual family members manage painful emotions in a similar way to what a mental health professional provides in therapy. Families that can turn to one another in times of great stress find that they are able to navigate even the most destructive storms in adaptive ways rather than choosing maladaptive responses such as numbing, distancing, or avoiding the associated painful feelings (Johnson, 2019). Families with secure attachments between members operate with communication that is direct, open, and honest with clear information, open emotional expression of the entire range of feelings, and utilizing active and collaborative problem-solving (Walsh, 2016).

Characteristics of Resilient Children:

- Social/adaptable temperament/empathy
- Strong cognitive abilities/able to redirect thoughts
- Effective emotional and behavioral regulation skills
- Positive view of self
- Overall positive outlook/optimistic
- Positive relationships with adults/teachers
- Sense of meaning in life/faith
- Characteristics valued by society and self
- Talents, humor, appearance

The military lifestyle comes with ongoing separations between family members and along with these separations come repetitive disruptions in family relationships and stability in family life. The repeated and often lengthy separations due to military demands for trainings and deployments can challenge even the strongest attachment bonds in family life. In addition to the cumulative nature of the quantity of time spent apart in military families, there is also often the added stress about the quality of many of these separations, particularly if they are to combat zones, hazardous duty stations, or higher-risk training situations. The combination of the significant quantity of time apart mixed together with the quality of that time often infused with risk for serious illness, injury, and/or death place military families at high risk for disruptions in the attachment bonds of family members. Efforts to strengthen the attachment bonds in military families should be made before, during, and after deployment separations in an ongoing manner to prevent harm to the overall functioning of the family system. Prevention can be done in terms of assessing the attachment bonds on a routine basis similar to health screenings. Attachment bonds that are strong between family members lead to healthy responses to stress and crisis among all members and prevent situations of family dissolution as a result. When family members are able to turn inward to each other for comfort in times of great emotional distress, they have more positive interactions in the home, and are less likely to respond behaviorally with maladaptive coping strategies such as evidenced in withdrawals, avoidance, and/or dysfunctional aggression misplaced onto the family system.

One of the therapeutic treatments targeted on facilitating development attachment between a child and parent is attachment-focused family therapy (Hughes, 2007). During this intervention, the family therapist will monitor the child's emotional state and comment on it out loud to facilitate this interaction by role modeling to the parent ways to strengthen the attachment bond (Hughes, 2007). The goals for this treatment are focused on what are known as "attunement behaviors" for the child and include the following: increasing the child's ability to engage in eye contact and ability to tolerate the parent's physical touch; increasing the child's ability to read and understand the parent's facial gestures; and improving the child's ability to self-moderate their physical responses to their environment and to stress. The therapist teaches the parent how to interact with the child in these areas through therapeutic play and then pulls away from the intervention to allow the parent–child dyad to work on these goals. Attunement behaviors are some of the most accurate behavioral predictors of the quality of the attachment bonds that are operating between family members at any given point in time in families. Assessments of attachment are easily viewed by focusing on the attunement behaviors that a child signals to his or her parent and include the following: eye contact that is tolerated and maintained for a period of time that can be measured by family members easily; the presence of "shared smiles" and "shared laughter" between family members, especially in the presence of eye contact; and the degree to which appropriate physical touch is tolerated and encouraged (reciprocally) between family members. Family sessions can include games as simple as the "thumb wrestling game" between family members that facilitates attachment through physical touch, emotional attunement, warmth, shared smiles, and laughter.

A similar intervention for improving the parent–child relationship bond is filial play therapy that focuses on increasing parental empathy and parental acceptance of the child which in turn then allows the child to be able to adjust to stress in healthier ways (Rennie & Landreth, 2000). The core concept in filial play therapy (with a parent and their child) is that when a child expresses feelings through play, without losing status in the eyes of their parents, the child's anxiety diminishes. Since adjustment difficulties in childhood are often associated with instability in interpersonal relationships in the family, the opportunity to strengthen these relationships and attachment ties helps the child feel validated, valued, and able to master feelings rather than deny or distort them. The child experiences the parent in a new manner and begins to feel a sense of self-worth through the eyes of their parent who assumes the role of being unconditionally understanding. The child's parent becomes their greatest ally in the process and in doing so, takes away parental resistance. Improvements have been demonstrated in the parent–child relationship due to the combination of focused attention on the child (2x/week) from a person who holds great significance and who clarifies miscommunications or cognitive distortions the child may be holding onto about the parent's risk levels and overall family life.

Family therapy with military families might include military-related themes such as toy soldiers, to facilitate and communicate feelings around deployments and provide an opportunity to correct misconceptions to be resolved if they are guiding children's behaviors. In addition to this, dinosaurs or soft dart guns allow for expression of feelings of aggression. For the exploration of caregiving, dependency, and attachment needs, baby bottles, dolls, and toy food facilitate such discussions around nurturance. Dollhouses, figures, toy furniture to explore family issues and communicate any family life incidents that may have happened while a child's parent was away from home or on a deployment should be included in the room. Simple childhood games such as ring toss, building blocks, and toy money facilitate the expression of mastery, competency, and cooperation in treatment sessions. In assessing the nature of the parent–child relationship, a family therapist working with military families will be able to gain great insights by taking a full description of the attachment behaviors prior to a stressful event such as a deployment separation. In doing so, they would assess for breaches or disruptions in the attachment that were evident prior to the stressful situation to be able to better understand how the attachment was influenced by the stress. In order to gain a full understanding of the relationship, questions that focus on the attachment are helpful to illustrate the strength of the attachment prior to the deployment. The following questions clarify with the caregiver, and/or both parents if present, what their unique perspectives are in relation to the family. and could be included in the assessment.

- How easy or difficult was it to get the child to brush teeth, pick up toys, etc.?
- How easily is affection demonstrated between family members and in dyad?
- How did the child respond in the past to bids for love and caring including smiles, reaching out for physical touch/hugs, eye contact, and parental requests for attunement?

An attachment assessment that reveals certain absent or negative attunement behaviors might address the following situations:

- Angry outbursts (in the home or at child's school);
- One or both parents being left out/not included in child's life;
- Irritable defiance to adult requests;
- Subtle, repeated manipulations;
- Lack of clear communications (verbal or non-verbal) with one or both parents;
- Parent feels angry, overwhelmed, or puzzled by child's reactions to reunions;
- Poor eye contact with parents;

- Avoidance by child of attempts at physical contact (hugs);
- Few shared smiles and/or little reciprocity to parent's overtures to connect, may even physically turn away from parent.

Solution-Focused Brief Therapy for Families

Solution-focused brief therapy (SFBT) is an ideal fit with the military culture, ethos, and perspectives on health, strength, and overcoming challenges through fitness, and resiliency. The focus on solutions rather than problems in this therapy encourages clients to identify what they would like their lives to look like rather than what is bothering them or creating stress in their lives at the time they seek counseling. In a reversal of many traditional psychotherapeutic treatment approaches that keep clients focused on problems, sessions focus on strengths and coping skills that have proven effective for them in the past. Rather than taking a medically centered approach where symptoms are viewed as evidence of a disease or a pathological condition, this strengths-based approach encourages clients to create behaviors that are based on a healthy adaptation to a situation that was, in fact, stressful.

Solution-focused brief therapy is a future-oriented model of psychotherapy treatment that focuses on strengthening resiliency rather than trying to understand what went wrong in one's past when someone was not resilient. The therapy does not focus on finding reasons why a client or family may be vulnerable and there is no search for someone to blame for times of stress. SFBT is in line with the concepts of positive psychology, based on collaborative and integrated efforts between client and therapist, to find solutions to the stressful situations in their lives, rather than origins for the stressful situations. SFBT employed by behavioral health treatment providers focuses on finding the exceptions to the problems that they are experiencing. One of the mottos used in SFBT is that "the exception is the solution." This simple guiding principle for the therapy aims to build psychological resilience by searching for coping skills that have been proven to work for the individual or family in stressful situations. In one of the first sessions of SFBT, the client or family will be asked to answer in detail the "miracle question" to elicit a description of what clients want more of in their lives rather than what they want to get rid of that is often the focus of therapy that is not strengths-based. A regular part of the sessions in SFBT is for clients to rate, scale, and measure the things that are bothering them and those that are working well for them in their lives on a scale from 1–10. These rating scales are present in sessions repeatedly so that client and therapist can mutually assess the client's progress in reaching their stated goals. The therapist takes a break during SFBT sessions and returns to offer a positive summary of specifics in the client or family's life. Following this positive summary, the therapist offers suggestions for behaviors outside the therapy session, framed in terms of these merely being "experiments" to see what happens with a shift in behavior or a changed perspective (de Shazer & Berg, 1997).

The focus of SFBT is not on what is going wrong in a client's life, but rather, in finding exceptions to the problems that lie in the client's competencies and abilities to succeed in those areas. In SFBT, the therapist will ask what was different in a person's life when things went well in that area and what a family wants it to be like rather than what they don't want in their lives. Metaphors are used to elicit which behaviors will be used/increased in the future instead of treatment goals that are focused on decreasing the current problematic behaviors. A stressful situation often arises with the notification of a PCS to a location that was unfamiliar to a military family who also heard about difficulties at that location especially if those involved school-related issues for children. The service member requested a different location but his request was denied, so he accepted that they would be moving to the base, and he adapted to the upcoming move. The military spouse, however, had not come to accept the move and worried constantly about the children's well-being. Her anxiety increased as she imagined "worst case scenarios" that included them losing a year of academic work, not fitting in socially with the other children there, and being bullied as a result. The couple began having arguments because the spouse believed that they "needed to do something" about the situation and the service member believed that they already had when he attempted to make a change but was denied. They were stuck in their abilities to join forces because they both had different perceptions of the situation that was preventing them from adapting to it together as a team. A solution-focused approach would identify how the couple wanted to interact with each other rather than focus on how they didn't want to interact. The couple would have to create the life they wanted without the problematic situation in it, and in this case that would mean that they were unified in their views about the upcoming move to the new location. They would visualize interacting with one another in ways that supported one unified view/perception for them both and would be encouraged to think of times they might have done something similar in the past. If they had done something similar together, that would be the exception to the problem, and the exception would be framed as the solution for them. They would think back to a time early in their marriage such as when their first child was a toddler and wouldn't sleep in his own bed at night. At that time, they had brainstormed solutions together and came up with a nightly routine that included all of his most comforting rituals such as finding the big dipper in the glow-in-the-dark stars on his wall and a bedtime story after a cup of warm milk. The couple would be able to laugh together at how easy that situation appeared to them now with ten years of parenting since then. This "long view" of having solved parenting stress in the past together as a team allows a couple to come together again and brainstorm things they would do together if any of their worries came true.

Trauma-Focused Family Therapy

Therapists working with veterans and military-connected families need to have a firm grasp on the theoretical framework that makes up trauma-informed care in order to provide effective treatment that does no harm to their clients. Trauma-informed care is a stage-based treatment where the therapy moves to the next stage when, and only when, the client is ready for it to move there. Given the combination of the military lifestyle

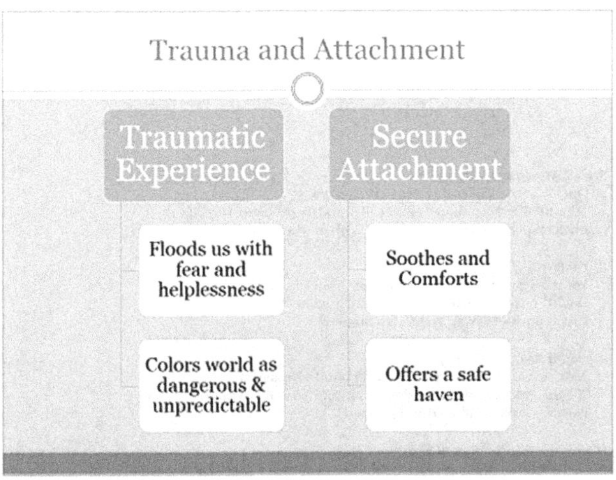

Figure 6.3 Trauma and attachment

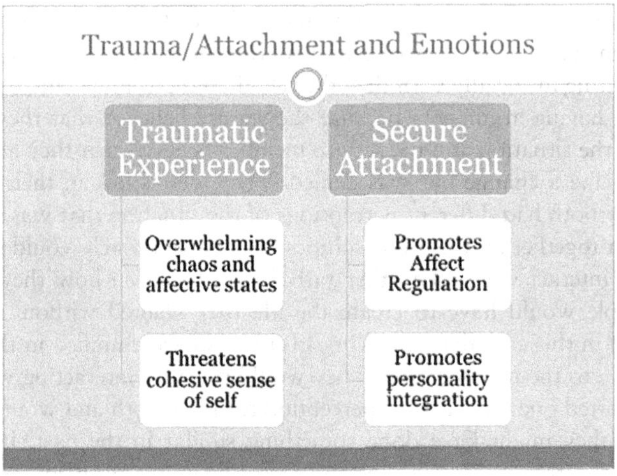

Figure 6.4 Trauma/attachment and emotions

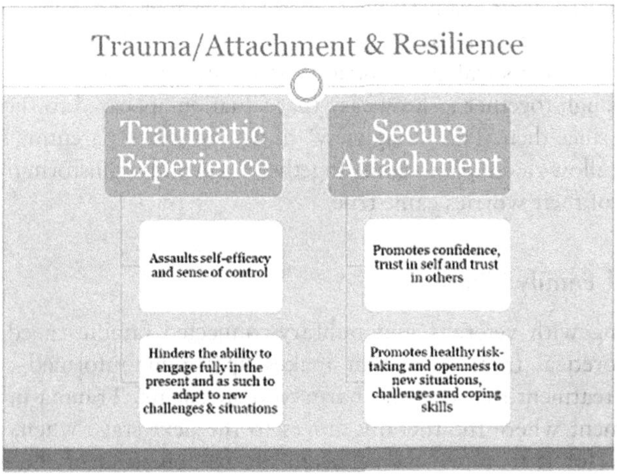

Figure 6.5 Trauma/attachment and resilience

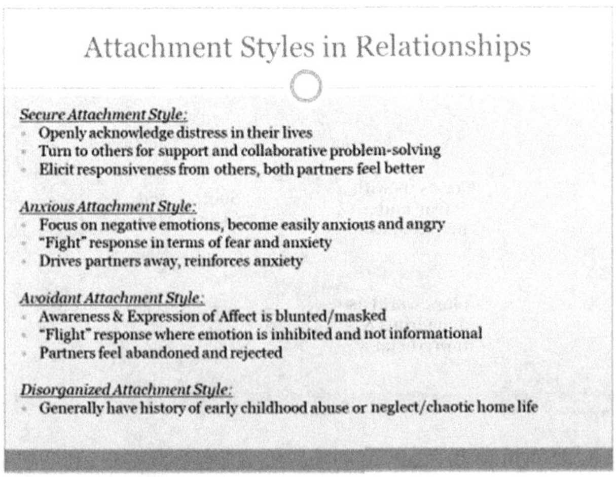

Figure 6.6 Attachment styles in relationships (Bowlby & Ainsworth, 2013)

with training missions and deployments that can involve threats to safety, and the associated need for establishing trust in relationships, therapists working with military families need to take an approach that is based on trauma-informed care at all times. A military-connected client or family does not need to have a history or diagnosis of trauma in order for the treatment lens to be one that has a trauma perspective to all interventions. Since one of the most pernicious effects stemming from trauma is a shattered belief in safety and trust in relationships, a trauma-informed care model focuses on strengthening attachment bonds in significant relationships. Figures 6.3–6.6 include the effects of trauma on resiliency, and recovery from posttraumatic stress, without the presence of the protective factor of secure attachments in significant family relationships.

Trauma impacts family functioning and relationships in multiple ways that have roots in three core areas of interpersonal functioning: affect regulation and expression; information processing; and the quality of communication between family members. The negative impact in these three areas challenges the attachment bonds and often results in disruptions in the stability of the attachments and relationships. Attachments that are secure and stable are protective against stress as they soothe the nervous system and allow individuals to manage overwhelming affects and be able to express and share their internal emotional states. Traumatic stress causes individuals to selectively attend to information in their environment in attempts to limit future danger and create safety as the world has proven to be unsafe to them. Information processing in the presence of traumatic stress can become rigidly fixed to support the changed perceptions of the world and relationships being unsafe and the self being vulnerable as a result.

Traumatic stress from combat that lingers in family life results in a heightened state of tension for all family members and shifts in role functioning and attachment security occurs as a result. The resiliency process of open and honest communication becomes frozen by the unpredictability of a home environment that is filled with traumatic stress reactions. Traumatic stress reactions often result in family members making accommodations for these reactions and difficulties regulating distance and closeness between family members. In terms of parenting, affect regulation problems that accompany traumatic stress can lead children to become confused about whether their parents can provide safety in the home as they witness accommodations being made for stress reactions. Role reversals may occur if children believe that they are better equipped to manage the environment and perceive themselves to be more in control of their own internal emotional states than their parents. Children with parents who have traumatic stress may grow up paying close attention to their environments and easily assume the role of caregiver if parents are experiencing out-of-control emotional states. These role changes often occur when the needs of the parents take priority over the needs of the children in ways that are rarely communicated or discussed collaboratively to ensure the safety, stability, and predictability of family life.

Cognitive Processing Therapy

Similar to the scaling questions found in SFBT, rating scales are utilized as a part of cognitive processing therapy, which has been adapted for combat veterans and widely utilized as one of the key manualized treatments currently offered to veterans at the V.A. for PTSD. Cognitive processing therapy (CPT) is a 12-session cognitive behavior therapy that is an evidence-based psychotherapy for PTSD considered a first-line treatment for service members and veterans diagnosed with PTSD. CPT is based on the social cognitive theory of PTSD that focuses on how the traumatic event is constructed cognitively, construed, and coped with by a person who is trying to regain a sense of mastery and control in their life (Resick et al., 2006). This treatment reports that there is a large drop in symptoms when assimilation of the trauma is occurring, often around the 5th or 6th session, assisted by written narratives and cognitive therapy that focuses on the trauma itself. This treatment utilizes evidence-based scales to measure PTSD symptoms and symptoms of depression (if co-existing) on a weekly basis as part of the manualized treatment. While both CPT and SFBT have similar goals, the main difference is in the paradigm used in these theories as the lens utilized in SFBT is on what works for the client and in CPT on what does not work for the client.

The focus in CPT is cognitive in nature as the very painful experience of living with unresolved trauma is associated with negative shifts in the individual's cognitive beliefs about oneself, others, and safety in the world. Clients engaged in CPT treatment identify situations that are problematic in their lives and create their own scales based on their own personal "subjective units of distress" for situations that trigger posttraumatic stress reactions on a scale of 0–100. In CPT, the client confronts these situations, tackling them in progressive order from the least bothersome to the most bothersome. The goals of CPT include reducing the symptoms of posttraumatic stress reactions through reducing avoidance behaviors that interfere in one's life and leave someone unable to engage in the identified activities of daily living. The focus includes challenging what are identified as maladaptive ways of thinking, also known as cognitive distortions or misperceptions, that have been constructed internally following a traumatic event that contribute to unhealthy patterns of behavior. The aim of CPT is to shift the trauma-influenced cognitive perceptions to more adaptive, healthier ones that will then influence behavioral outcomes in daily life to ones that are more positive and reduce the avoidance, intrusion, and arousal symptoms that accompany unresolved traumatic stress. Clients who have depression and other serious mental health issues need to engage with caution in CPT and all of the cognitive behavioral therapies as the use of phrases such as "distorted thinking, misperceptions, and maladaptive patterns" can reinforce negative self-perceptions. Treatment that monitors for negative shifts in self-perceptions on a regular basis ensures that this is not happening in the treatment process and serves to keep clients proceeding in a safe manner while they engage in therapy that is extremely difficult in cognitive, social, and emotional ways.

Solution-Focused Brief Therapy (Case Example)

A dual-military family engaged in SFBT shortly after the news of an upcoming deployment of one of the parents and the couple had started having disagreements over how they would manage the separation in terms of childcare issues. The service member who would be staying at home believed that she needed more support for the younger children in the family and didn't want to assume that the teenage son would be willing or able to provide this support. The couple identified specific situations in the past where similar challenges were overcome without arguments and because family members communicated directly with one another, everyone got along and even had fun in the process despite the stressful situation. The couple identified goals they would like to see more of in family life to meet the current challenging situation that brought them into treatment that included: more positive interactions in family life, more communication of positive thoughts and feelings in daily life, more fun, and more instances where family members would "just go with the flow" of family life. The couple was encouraged by the therapist that since they did this once, they had the capacity to do it again. The couple identified that they got along better and solved problems more collaboratively when they did not take a position and hold onto it in rigid fashion so the therapist gave them "homework" around this goal. The therapist suggested that whenever either member of the couple wanted to hold onto a position that they try an experiment of "going with the flow" instead and just see what happened as a result. The couple tried this and were both surprised to find how easy it was to change a pattern of negative interactions when committing to the change was not a part of the treatment. The idea of trying something different just as an experiment to see what happened, allowed the couple to see that it worked, and they both felt positive about the way they were interacting in family life. The couple did the same thing with open emotional expression in their communications and they just tried behaviors to see what happened. They discovered that they were relieved and surprised by the results. The family was able to increase their collaborative problem-solving skills and experienced more positive interactions than they had previously. There were fewer conflicts and they found solutions that worked for them as a family. In addition to these goals, the therapist added a goal for strengthening the attachments with the children in the family through increasing attunement behaviors. The parents agreed to "just try it" once to see how it went and found that making eye contact, sharing smiles, and sharing laughter with their children increased everyone's overall sense of lightness in the family. Positivity became contagious as the more the family experienced it, the more often they sought out opportunities to have this happen again, and again, in repeated fashion.

Part 3

Post-Deployment Resiliency

"Assessing the Effects of the Storm"

7 Posttraumatic Stress in Military Family Life

Resiliency and Stress

The significant process during this phase is understood to be similar to a puzzle piece that was taken out of a finished puzzle, had life-changing experiences and can no longer fit into the space that it once occupied in that puzzle. It is easy for most people to understand that a military service member will change from the experience of going to war. What often comes as a surprise to many people, however, is that military family members will change as well from the experience. There is a common misperception that the family at home remains stable and constant during a deployment separation, and while this may happen for some families, it is typically not the reality for most families. The experience of sending an immediate family member to war is one that is highly impactful to family life and to all family members in their own unique ways. The family may relate to one another differently than they did before the separation and may react to changes in one another based on a combination of factors including their perceptions, developmental level, personal histories of coping with stress, and any challenges present in daily life. The experience of a family member being at war brings with it the ever-present reality that that person could die at any time during the separation and not return home or back to the family. While there are countless efforts taken on the part of the service member and the military to prevent this from happening, the family can do little in this area other than try not to upset or distract the service member while on a combat deployment. This reality often adds to the stress experienced by family members feeling powerless to protect their loved one at war. Military families must tolerate very difficult and painful emotions on a daily basis such as high levels of anxiety together with disempowerment and lack of control over the family's present and future situations.

Service members, spouses, children, parents, siblings, and other significant loved ones change during wartime separations, particularly if it had been lengthy or extended, and especially if the family lacks social support or has negative experiences including interpersonal violence, racism, or other forms of oppression. When the family reunites following a wartime deployment, the many adaptations that family members have made to cope with the situation will appear in family relationships, attachment bonds, and overall levels of familial functioning. Individual family members who took on caregiving roles for other family members may have done so in a crisis orientation and coped with the situation by suppressing feelings that were distressing or painful. When the crisis is over, family members often expect to return to previous ways of functioning in the family as a system, however for some families, the crisis continues in a new way and often even worsens following a deployment.

Family members will react to changes in one another and the family as a whole based on the magnitude of the demands during the reintegration period as well as their own

DOI: 10.4324/9781003438229-11

personal histories of coping, adapting, and managing stressful situations. There are significant changes in children that have developed in age and maturity levels with communication challenges that need to be resolved. The family system as a whole now needs to adapt to these individual changes and changes in interpersonal relationships and the home environment. As most life transitions bring up some degree of difficulty and confusion surrounding changes taking place, family members need to be able to discuss the situation as well as their thoughts and feelings so the family can adapt and move on to their next chapter.

Family members need to possess the psychological and social skills for open and honest communication to be able to discuss the changes that are taking place around them. In order to do this, there needs to be trust between members, and in order to have trust, the family must have security in their attachments to one another. Children who have grown up cognitively and developmentally during a deployment may have new questions, feelings, and changes in the ways that they perceive, relate, and interact with both of their parents. Children who move into the developmental period of adolescence, for example, are likely to experience shifts in their thinking that move them into more abstract ways of seeing the world and they may question behaviors in their parents that they never questioned previously. A young child who was a toddler when a parent left for a lengthy deployment may have entered school and developed more social skills and concrete ways of thinking. School-aged children typically employ ways of thinking and interacting that allow for healthy and appropriate suppression of emotions in order to complete the tasks of this stage of development. Communication among all family members needs to consider childhood developmental shifts when discussing changes in the family environment. As children are developing all the time, they may be surprised to see changes in their parents at the same time, especially if these cause anxiety for children who were relying on parental stability in order to make those developmental shifts. The absence of open and honest communication to clarify changes in relationships, attachments, and in their parents can easily cause behavioral regressions or an inability to take the next developmental step for many children.

Family organization is important in resiliency in the period that follows a deployment separation because it provides the stability that family rituals and routines offer to children in the midst of such a major life transition. The family needs to maintain a sense of stability that is best achieved through having a sense of healthy leadership by parents who respect boundaries and role model collaborative problem solving through open and honest conversations about difficult topics. The concept that there exist solutions to all of life's challenges and problems is necessary and adds a layer of comfort to all family members in transition. The sense of stability, continuity, and dependability on the part of the parents provides the flexibility that children need to be able to adapt to the changes in the family system. Parents need to mobilize social supports and community networks to be able to maintain financial security during transition times and achieve a healthy balance of work and family life as a result. In terms of belief systems following a deployment, families need to maintain a sense of hopefulness that any adversity will be managed through the strengths inherent in the family system. Resilient families tend to view adversity as a collective challenge that the family will meet together with values based on a higher purpose than individual family members' goals and happiness. Resilience in families is relational in nature and adversity is managed within that context by the strengths of the relationships. Resilient families operate as a collective and the collectivist mentality is one that places the group over individual needs, wants, or goals or taking care of oneself if it means the group will suffer as a result.

Social support has been documented to decrease symptoms of posttraumatic stress in combat veterans after returning home from war among many other health and mental health-related improvements. In an effort to increase social support for the current generation of veterans and military families, the National Academies of Sciences, Engineering, and Medicine recommended that the U.S. Department of Defense increase civilian understanding of the military population, address stereotypes, and clarify misinformation in the public sector (2019). The recommendations included the need for increased awareness among the civilian population of military culture and the experiences of military children to strengthen social support and build a stronger sense of belonging across communities. Social support is a protective factor in resiliency for veterans returning from home following wartime military service. The time that WWI and WWII veterans spent together on boats returning home, coupled with the pervasive community support and vast numbers of veterans at home, was positive and helpful in terms of managing what would otherwise have been overwhelming stress if experienced in community-based isolation.

Racism and Military Service

Military families who experience racism and other forms of discrimination have additional layers of risk that can make family adjustment to stress a more difficult and challenging process to navigate. Throughout the 19th century, the United States fought multiple wars against Native American tribes, more than were fought against foreign countries (Treuer, 2019). In tandem with these wars, federal policies including the "Indian Removal Act" (1830) and the "General Allotment Act" (1887) that displaced Native Americans from their homes and lands onto reservations, resulted in ongoing cycles of poverty. Thousands of Native American children went to residential schools funded by the federal government and were forbidden to speak tribal languages, practice their religion, or wear traditional clothing. These strict, military-style boarding schools produced thousands of students who received extensive vocational training and who volunteered to join the military during WWI, most of whom as infantry soldiers, despite years of vocational training for other military occupational specialties (Treuer, 2019). The author reports that approximately 150 Sioux died by the U.S. Cavalry in the 1890 massacre at Wounded Knee and have struggled to be resilient through collective resistance to oppressive forces both locally and in wider communities historically.

According to Koehlmoos et al. (2022), the majority of racial and ethnic minority service members are in enlisted ranks (almost one-third of all active-duty personnel) and 25% in the rank of officer. Systemic and individual experiences with racism and other forms of discrimination and oppression play a significant role in military family life, coping strategies, and adjustment to the stress of a deployment. Taking the "Double ABCX" theoretical model of family adaptation to stress of McCubbin and Patterson (1983), a family's unique stressors combine with the family's resources (financial, educational, formal and informal support networks) and perceptions/meaning that the family gives to the stress. If the loss of the service member in a family to a deployment negatively affects the family's ability to manage situations of daily living, or causes the family to perceive that they are less able to manage certain situations, these will place the family at risk for negative outcomes in the adjustment. One such example of this is systemic racism that may leave a family to be less safe without the presence of a service member who may have mediated instances such as micro-aggressions or violence perpetrated against family members. A military family's experiences of racism, targeted violence, oppression, and/or discrimination in their communities, schools, work, relationships, and military lives will all negatively affect the family's overall adjustment to a deployment situation.

Racial and ethnic minority service members have historically been subject to discrimination both during military service and upon returning home from war. The inequalities experienced in American civilian life were present for military veterans throughout history and included multiple unjust practices of segregation and voting rights. Promises made for access to home ownership, business loans, and higher education went unfulfilled as these entry points for upward social mobility were denied by states' rights and private colleges who did not admit and/or forced out non-White students who had already been admitted. The first non-White military Army regiment was formed in 1775, comprised of Black slaves and "freedmen" to aid in the Revolutionary War, and these soldiers were often treated in demeaning, racist ways by their White peers and commanding officers. In addition to these soldiers, reinforcements from Mexico, Cuba, Venezuela, and the Philippines fought to assist the colonists in the Revolutionary War against the British as well as Native Americans who often fought for both sides to preserve their land ownership (Yamada, Atuel, & Weiss, 2013; Coll, Weiss, & Metal, 2013). Most of the Black soldiers who had been slaves of the colonists before the war remained in slavery following the war. Native American warriors who entered the war to keep their land in return for fighting for the colonies remained on their land for a few decades but lost these tribal lands in the 1800s in multiple violent wars with the U.S. military. In addition to mistreatment during their service in the military, promises of freedom, land preservation, pathways to citizenship, and upward social mobility often never materialized for racial and ethnic minority veterans following their military service.

In World War II, 1.2 million African Americans served in combat forces and returned from the war to the same socioeconomic discrimination and racist violence experienced before military service despite their sacrifices overseas. Black and other ethnic/minority veterans struggled to get hired for well-paying jobs and encountered segregation that continued systemically throughout American culture at home. These veterans endured targeted brutality, especially while wearing their military uniforms, when they returned home despite having served in heavy combat missions. The 761 Tank Battalion was the first Black division to face ground combat in Europe as they joined Patton's Third Army in France in November 1944, helped to liberate 30 towns under Nazi control, and spent 183 days in combat including in the Battle of the Bulge. The Tuskegee Airmen were an all-Black fighter pilot group trained at Tuskegee Institute in Alabama whose service included escorting bombers over Italy and Sicily and these pilots flew in approximately 1,600 combat missions during the war, risking their lives in military combat on a daily basis, and returned to experience violent and widespread racism in their own country.

President Franklin D. Roosevelt signed the G.I. Bill into law in 1944 to prevent mass unemployment among veterans and a post-war economic depression that included tuition assistance in higher education, job placement, and federally subsidized bank loans to buy new homes and to start new businesses. The N.A.A.C.P. and other civil rights groups encouraged Blacks to enlist in the military so they could receive G.I. Bill benefits, however, the G.I. Bill failed to propel Black veterans into the middle class in the numbers that it did for White veterans and there is scarce data recorded on the experience for other ethnic minority groups. These benefits resulted in 86% of professional/skilled jobs going to White veterans and 92% of unskilled jobs going to Black veterans. Many Black veterans were denied access to a college education, largely relegated to vocational programs, with 28% of White veterans going to college on the G.I. Bill compared with 12% of Black veterans. Of that 12% of Black veterans who went on to attend higher education, 90% of them attended historically Black colleges mainly in the South that were under-funded and had limited resources. Veteran enrollments at historically Black colleges skyrocketed from 29,000 in 1940 to 73,000 in 1947 and an estimated 20,000 to 50,000 Black veterans were turned away due to limited capacity at these institutions.

Home ownership creates equity, an investment in the future, and wealth for the next generation. Black and other minority veterans did not have the opportunity to create a future generation with economic security due to the racist policies and practices operating throughout many of the systemic institutions in the United States. The G.I. Bill guaranteed mortgages for homes, farms, and businesses and data from the post-war years reported that 67% of Whites had home ownership while 40% of Blacks had home ownership. Small-business loans from the Department of Veterans Affairs were often denied to Black veterans and a 1947 survey of 13 cities in Mississippi found that of the total of 3,229 home loans given to Veterans in that year, only two went to African American veterans. The history of systemic racism impacted racial and ethnic minority service members and their families throughout history and was clearly evidenced in state and federal policies around rolling out the G.I. Bill benefits that were promised to veterans to entice them to join military service. In addition to the countless injuries, deaths, and sacrifices of Black and minority veterans who honorably served their country in the military, government promises were unfilled, family resiliency was threatened, and the opportunity for upward social and economic mobility often never materialized. Although the G.I. Bill is no longer the same as it was in 1947, the societal impact of systemic racism continues in pervasive ways to make upward mobility one of the most challenging aspects of American life for the majority of non-White citizens. Black and minority veterans have documented historical and systemic racism and racist practices in the military that have kept most Black and minority service members out of the highest ranks of the military due to glass ceilings from entrenched systemic practices.

Being limited to lower-ranking positions as service members comes with lower levels of income and status in the military ranks, which then leads to later decreased income and retirement benefits from these lower levels. The link between service-connected medical retirements and systemic racism is an issue needing more research to inform military policy on uncovering systemic bias in the military that leads service members toward discharge from service or to a military medical retirement that comes with increased financial benefits. Many advocacy groups call for military-connected communities to keep track of service-connected disability ratings in the post-9/11 era to determine the connections between systemic racism, disability ratings, and benefits received by minority veterans. In addition to systemic racism, issues related to discrimination based on other markers of identity (including sex, gender, and sexual orientation) could be kept track of in order for service members who served to receive equity in benefits they are entitled to as a result of their military service.

Traumatic Stress in Military Families

Returning home from war is a difficult process for many veterans to navigate as they leave behind the experience of living on a constant high level of alert and danger to return to family life in peacetime. Although military communities hold an event for the return of service members, this is not typically held among the civilian community. Some Indigenous peoples have historically held ceremonies involving drums for the symbolic release of psychological pain and present-day ceremonies may involve veterans as they are believed to know the "weight" of life and death (Treuer, 2019). A practice exists among certain Native American tribes for warriors to receive the healing that comes when one's community recognizes the reintegration experience as a collective wound to all members, even non-warriors, and accepts responsibility together for sending the warrior to fight on their behalf. When warriors return from war, they are still in the warrior mindset, which by the sheer nature of it places distance in their civilian social relationships situated in a civilian mindset and value system. This distance makes reintegration difficult because warriors need to shift their value system back to civilian values and a civilian mindset. Warriors who participate in rituals designed to assist them in this process are vulnerable in the presence of community members to allow feelings that may include regret, shame, guilt, remorse, and/or other feelings to emerge. Tears wiped away from the warrior represent permission to return to civilian ways of life and values. The transition away from the warrior mindset and value system is assisted through this ritual and creates a bridge that returns the warrior to civilian status. This process acknowledges deep, sometimes painful, feelings that result from wartime participation and allows the burden of these to exist collectively among civilian peers in the community as well as within the warrior him or herself.

One of the least researched and documented areas of family functioning and impact on family life following military deployments is the experience and the well-being of the military spouse. Military spouses have reported a pervasive and disturbing lack of information from both the military and civilian communities about how to manage living with posttraumatic stress reactions in a veteran family member. The overwhelming majority of studies to date do not concern spouses of U.S. service members but rather spouses in other countries. One study with spouses of U.S. Army National Guard service members found that the spouses experienced symptoms that were along the same four domains of criteria as their veteran spouses (re-experiencing, avoidance, emotional numbing, and hyper-arousal) as measured with a modified version of the military checklist for traumatic stress symptoms (Bjornestad et al., 2014). In this study, the spouses reported secondary traumatic responses in the following descending order: avoiding events and circumstances that could trigger memories; feeling isolated; experiencing few emotional sensations; being extraordinarily aware or vigilant; avoiding thoughts, conversations, or emotions; problems staying engaged; difficulties with anger management; feeling nervous or anxious; distressed when reminded; loss of interest in leisure activities; physiological reactions; unexpectedly reliving; recurring nightmares; recurring distressing recollections of spouse's stressful military experience; difficulties with sleep; believing they might have a reduced future; and difficulties recalling certain aspects of significance.

Among the veterans in the study, approximately half reported symptoms of hyper-arousal (difficulties with sleep, concentration, easily startled, on guard, and feeling irritable or having angry outbursts) and feeling distant or cut off from other people, and almost half of the veterans reported that they felt that they had changed as a result of the deployment (Bjornestad et al., 2014). In addition to the symptoms that were reported (some spouses left answers blank possibly out of stigma or fear of reprisals for the spouse's career), the severity of these were correlated with the severity of the veteran's symptoms. As the veteran spouse's posttraumatic stress scores increased, the at-home spouse's secondary traumatic stress scores increased. The veterans in the study were more likely to report hyper-arousal symptoms than symptoms in the other three domains, which the authors attribute to a possible link of the perception of these symptoms being less disabling, more expected, or normative than the other areas (re-experiencing, avoidance, and emotional numbness). The question was left from these conclusions of which of these domains might be perceived as the most disabling or damaging to both the veteran's military career and to military family life. As perceptions influence coping and collaborative family problem solving, military couples would benefit from comparing their individual perceptions of which of these domains impacts relationships and family functioning.

A qualitative study conducted with female spouses of active-duty Marines sheds light on some of these answers from the spouse's perceptions of living with a combat veteran with posttraumatic stress (Temple et al., 2017). The results reported five themes: great unpredictability of daily life; the spouse had to take on different roles; the spouses felt unprepared to handle the symptoms and the stress; the spouses received different messages when trying to seek help for their husbands; and the wives wanted to send messages to other wives living with Marines with posttraumatic stress. The first theme reported was unpredictability that entered family life due to not knowing what mood the veteran spouse was going to be in when they walked through the door and spouses reported believing that they were living with two different people, never knowing which one was going to emerge at any given time. Some women reported that this anxiety bled into other areas of their lives including their careers and caused impairments in their occupational functioning as a result. In addition to their careers, spouses have also reported a generalized anxiety associated with living with a combat veteran as well as heightened anxiety and attempts to protect their children from their veteran partner's irritability, angry outbursts, unpredictable moods, and other stress reactions.

The second theme that emerged was that wives reported needing to assume new and unexpected roles in relation to their veteran spouse, including protector, caregiver, babysitter, and mother figure. These women described falling into these roles in attempts to prevent the veteran from having traumatic stress reactions in public or at work that would jeopardize their careers and family security as a result. They reported being on heightened alert at all times to make sure the veteran was not experiencing any reactions, and would pay close attention to signs of internal triggers in their husbands as well as external triggers in the environment. In addition to this constant behavior or keeping watch over their spouses, some of the women reported communicating what situations to avoid and when to stop drinking to their spouses to protect them from getting into trouble as a result of their stress reactions.

The third theme was that the women felt unprepared and uninformed by the military about how to manage and cope with posttraumatic stress in their veteran spouses. This lack of information led the wives to question their sanity as well as their relationships with their husbands. Many of the women believed that their husbands were engaging in destructive behaviors because of something that they had said or done and blamed themselves for the post-deployment conflicts in the marriages. The fourth theme involved getting mixed messages about what to do to get help as the military had constant messages about reaching out for help and not believing in a stigma. One woman was informed by other members of her husband's unit that no Marine should have PTSD from her husband's deployment because there was no traumatic event or firefight that would justify having PTSD. The response that some of the wives got from the military was that the spouses' cries for help didn't matter because service members have regular health assessments that screen for the presence of mental health symptoms and conditions. If the military assessed that the service member was fit for duty, then they were fit for duty, and the military unit and command would know if they were not. If a service member is having conflicts with a spouse that is generally considered a private matter unless it rises to a level that includes violence or impairs the service member's performance related to military occupational duties, tasks, and/or responsibilities. The last theme was that the wives wanted other wives to know that marital problems that appeared post-combat and in the presence of traumatic stress symptoms were not their fault. They wanted to send a clear message to other military spouses in similar situations that it is not their fault if their veteran spouse is drinking more alcohol, behaving more aggressively, isolating from friends/family, and lashing out in unpredictable ways: it is the fault of posttraumatic stress from combat. All the spouses described emotional pain, fear of their husbands, and fear of reaching out for help for themselves and their families.

Other messages reported were that spouses in these situations must have support if living with a veteran with traumatic stress; must know that they cannot change traumatic stress reactions on their own and that such reactions will not disappear without the veteran's involvement; and that providers who are willing and able to help need to be vocal about where they are due to the nature of the military ethos of tolerating pain leading to layers and layers of secrecy for military couples getting help when they are ready.

The avoidance symptoms of posttraumatic stress including numbing and withdrawal negatively impacts communication and impairs the flexibility in thinking necessary for collaborative problem-solving in intimate partner relationships. Spouses who attempt to maintain family stability by making accommodations for posttraumatic stress symptoms may unintentionally reinforce the stress symptoms and increase emotional dependence on them (Monson et al., 2009). Partners of combat veterans have reported that their efforts to protect their veteran spouse from posttraumatic stress triggers are often met with anger and resentment from the veterans, who perceived this behavior as controlling, and the spouses in turn became a new trigger as a result of the couple's maladaptation (Gerlock et al., 2014). Resilient couples in the same study communicated directly about the traumatic stress symptoms and the impact of those symptoms on the relationship as well as on the non-military spouse. This communication often included discussions about the veteran's military experiences on deployments that addressed any traumatic material head-on and thereby prevented the need for trauma-related avoidance. These resilient couples responded to the situation directly and did not allow for the secrecy that can be part of the warrior ethos. In having honest and open conversations, the resilient couples were also able to bridge the military versus civilian divide that can tear apart marital relationships where one spouse is non-military. Resilient partners reported setting clear boundaries regarding their responsibilities and self-care, identified specific coping strategies, and spoke of themselves as a unified team fighting together against the traumatic stress that was viewed as the enemy rather than the relationship itself.

Topics that may heavily influence family adaptation to stress following a military deployment may include traumatic incidents that were experienced or witnessed by the service member as well as the service member's perceptions and beliefs concerning them. If the deployment was during wartime, the service member may return home with feelings that can range from relief and happiness at being safe at home to sorrow and despair for lives that were lost and guilt that is associated with surviving a situation when others did not. Following the return from a deployment, there is ideally ample "dwell" time before returning to another deployment in order for the service member to be able to process their thoughts, feelings, and perceptions about the experience. When there is a lack of resolution about situations that may have occurred during a deployment, or unresolved adversity in family life afterwards, a family may gain a sense of relief from another separation. Although another deployment or training separation may offer relief, families that do not resolve questions and meet adversity by turning away from it are likely to experience new stressors in family life as a result. Families that turn away from adversity as a means for managing it may never get the chance to develop the skills together as a cohesive family system to make meaning out of the adversity and be able to understand it in a coherent family narrative. In situations such as these, individual family members are left on their own to make meaning out of crisis in isolation from the group narrative and are at risk for creating very diverse narratives that assign blame and causality to other family members. Isolated individual family narratives are often created with misinformation, misperceptions, and/or cognitive distortions based on a lack of clarifying information from other family members that can lead to splinters in familial attachment bonds.

The Warrior without a War

Any two people can experience the same traumatic incident and are likely to have very different posttraumatic responses based on a variety of issues. There are certain protective factors that influence whether an individual will remain in a heightened state of stress following trauma beyond a period of time that is adaptive in nature. There are also risk factors such as patterns of coping with stress in one's history that are likely to influence whether an individual's posttraumatic stress response will become chronic in nature. In addition to an individual's response to posttraumatic stress, there are certain adaptive responses that families can choose as ways of responding to its presence in family life.

The cumulative length of time spent in war-related deployments has been reported to have an increased negative impact on the post-deployment reintegration process for military families rather than providing some degree of immunity or relief from its effects. One study found that the longer the time spent in deployment separations (to Iraq and Afghanistan), the greater the probability of divorce among couples who did not expect changes in marital satisfaction and stress was present during the reintegration period (Negrusa & Negrusa, 2014). The study found that the presence of post-deployment stress symptoms in military families increased the divorce probability by 10–20% for Army enlisted service members and 50–75% among Army officers (Negrusa & Negrusa, 2014). Most of the military couples in the study reported believing that the experience of serving during war wouldn't impact the marital relationship or the couple's functioning following it. While the deployment experience itself was anticipated to be a destabilizing process to marital stability, it was one that most couples believed they would recover from and that marital stability would return. When marital stability did not return as anticipated, the attachments suffered, and the process can be viewed through the family adaptation to stress model described previously where perceptions and cognitive confusion was destabilizing to military couples and led to different interpretations and narratives of the situation.

These findings point to the need for increased communication among military couples in the periods before and during deployment separations as a way to prevent marital dissatisfaction from emerging unexpectedly following the post-deployment return to family life. In terms of prevention of marital strife and to increase family resiliency for families in the midst of deployment cycles, the military could offer trainings to service members and spouses prior to a deployment around this topic. It would seem that an overall increased awareness that changes will occur in couple functioning in the post-deployment phase of the cycle would be beneficial and easy to offer. The notion that family members will remain the same following a deployment separation appears to be a pervasive belief among many that would be an area to target to prevent marital dissatisfaction and family dissolution from happening as a result. Military service members, spouses, and families would have increased resiliency if changes in family life were normalized and to be expected post-deployment. The concept that all family members are going to change during a deployment separation would include the following areas: children are going to grow and mature developmentally; spouses are going to gain increased competency and occupy independent roles in the marriage; and service members are going to experience a range of situations from developing leadership skills and expertise in their military roles to experiencing challenging and/or traumatic situations. All family members will change. It is normal and it is to be expected. Resilient families need to have the tools to adapt to these changes as an interactive system to meet the demands of family life post-deployment to continue to function in healthy ways.

Significant events that threaten an individual's survival, whether by immediate assault to that person's life or by witnessing such a threat to another person's life are traumatic in nature and cause an internal psychological response as a result of that threat. The immediate response to a traumatic incident is typically a heightened level of stress during the incident that serves as a tool to survive the threat. When the immediate threat is over, however, this heightened acute stress lingers for a period of time to ensure that the threat is no longer present, that it will not return, and that there are no other threats present in the environment. This stress response is a normal and healthy adaptive response to a life-threatening situation. All traumatic situations are different and while every individual response is unique, there are common responses that emerge. The acute response to a traumatic incident may resolve itself in a relatively short period of time (days or weeks) as the individual makes sense of the danger and appraises its continued threat to survival. When this does not occur, the response lingers beyond what is necessary for survival, and becomes entrenched in daily life. If the traumatic experience is chronic or ongoing in nature, the stress response is an adaptive means for surviving and the response becomes habitual and chronic in nature. The posttraumatic response that lingers when the danger is no longer present often becomes maladaptive as the individual continues to respond in a heightened stress state on a regular basis as if they are still living in danger and fearful of being hurt and/or killed.

Instability and conflicts are also seen in the parent–child relationship post-deployment as a result of the destabilizing shock from the exit and return of the service member in the family system. Attachment security and posttraumatic stress are inexorably intertwined as the behaviors that lead to avoidance of social events negatively impact relationship functioning post-deployment for military children and families. In a military couple, when avoidance behaviors are evidenced, there is often a response on the part of family members to interrupt behavioral avoidance which often leads to conflicts in the family system and individual relationships within it. The dynamic of withdrawal and social avoidance and the family response of pursuing and demanding is one that families are often unaware is happening although often clear to outside observers such as extended family, friends, or neighbors. The unfortunate reality is that this observation is one that very few people are willing to make for fear of intruding into the privacy of the nuclear family. By the time a therapist is employed to offer this observation, it is often too late, as other ripple effects often occur in terms of related maladaptive coping responses to the loss of the marital satisfaction and damage that has occurred to family relationships and attachment security.

Many veterans with traumatic stress following deployments report great difficulty with reintegration into the family system and previous roles in the family and community due primarily to the arousal symptoms of the condition. The arousal symptoms of posttraumatic stress disorder are easily seen, experienced, and expressed as anger or reactions of impulsive rage when they come about unexpectedly. In the event that one family member has repeated reactions to triggers in the environment that are unpredictable, and continue in a chronic manner over time, it can lead a family to decrease their overall patterns of social engagement and interpersonal relationships with networks outside of the family system. The domino effect of having trait expressions of anger may be the result that families can become socially isolated at a time when social support is needed the most as it is widely helpful in the resolution of traumatic stress. Many families can experience feelings of depression throughout this process and family functioning can deteriorate without social support networks or community-based interventions aimed at increasing social engagement.

Social support is one of the most important resiliency factors in coping with situations of great distress and in the prevention of mental health symptoms and illness from developing. It has been known to reduce physiological reactivity to stress, lessen debilitating appraisals of threat in the environment, and to assist with the development of effective coping strategies. One study with older U.S. veterans who endured a high number of traumas in their lifetimes found that the majority who were psychologically resilient had reported increased social connectedness, community integration, and having a sense of purpose in life. Social ties through both formal and informal community networks created a sense of attachment security for many people who had experienced interrupted attachments in their lives that had resulted from trauma.

Full and Partial Posttraumatic Stress

There is a pressing need to discuss and develop treatments for veterans and their families who experience some, but not all, of the symptoms of PTSD and one study investigating this group found an intermediate level of impairment (Pietrzak & Cook, 2013). Veterans with partial PTSD report problems with their spouse/partner, difficulty connecting emotionally with their family, being unhappy with their job, not getting along with their co-workers, relating better to veterans than civilians, holding the belief that civilian friends do not understand them, and not having interests in common with their civilian friends. They also identified having relationship problems and work-related problems and wanting help for these problems.

The awareness that veterans with "partial PTSD or PTS" experience problems in health, work, and family functioning speaks to the need to reach this group who are likely to not be receiving crucial validation of their suffering that can be healing in creating new narratives. Military spouses and family members as well are denied a full and complete understanding of behavioral changes in their family system following deployments that are often provided to families of veterans diagnosed with full PTSD through the V.A. and programs that address it. Given that Partial PTSD is not a recognized diagnosis in the health care communities, it is not being identified as a condition during medical and mental health evaluations and during routine military health assessments and reassessments every year. Clinicians in the healthcare systems and veteran-connected communities may be underestimating the magnitude of impairment associated with partial PTSD in veterans from the wars in Iraq and Afghanistan, which may decrease mental health treatment-seeking in this population, negatively affect health and psychosocial functioning, and delay successful reintegration into civilian life (Pietrzak & Cook, 2013).

In addition to clinicians being unable to identify or name a cluster of behaviors seen in veterans that are below threshold for full PTSD diagnostic criteria, they are also unable as a result of this lack of knowledge, to correctly treat this group of veterans and their family members. One of the most significant results that comes from not naming or understanding a condition in an individual you are treating is that treatments aimed at other areas may not only be missing the target but could also potentially be damaging to the person. For example, someone who is being seen in mental health treatment for anger management issues or alcohol misuse may be experiencing partial PTSD and need treatment that targets these symptoms and would understand the anger and alcohol use in terms of mediating traumatic stress rather than something entirely different. Family functioning in light of partial PTSD would be understood differently as well and family members need to learn the skills and tools to manage traumatic stress in the home environment also. Families who understand the nature of behaviors in the family system have more tools to address the interpersonal dynamic of relationships and family functioning overall.

Secondary Traumatic Stress in the Family System

Traumatic triggers in the family system and home environment that cause automatic negative responses for one family member have cascading effects on all family members. As one member responds to internal and/or external reminders and cues of their own personal traumatic experience, patterns of behaviors emerge in familial relationships as other family members cope with these traumatic stress reactions (Figure 7.1). Families with an ill or injured family member will typically adjust their behaviors and interactions to maintain stability in the family and limit negative consequences to the overall integrity as a functioning system. In this way, family members collude (often non-verbally) to limit unpredictability, confusion, and chaos in the home environment by adjusting behaviorally. Posttraumatic stress in an adult family member has the potential to create a family system that is unstable due to the lack of predictability of daily life. Patterns of chronic, unpredictable posttraumatic stress reactions in family life can lead to secondary traumatic stress reactions as all family members respond to an environment that is not safe and predictable, but rather, chaotic and threatening or even dangerous in the worst situations. In addition to this, family members with their own personal histories of trauma are at risk for decreased resiliency during reintegration periods filled with posttraumatic stress as traumatic material that may have been dormant can easily resurface in the intersubjective nature of close family relationships. The combination of a close attachment bond with a family member experiencing chronic traumatic stress and an unpredictable home environment can cause secondary traumatic stress symptoms to emerge for family members as a result.

Research has documented the existence of transmission of traumatic stress among family members; most of it has been in an intergenerational pattern, and the need for more research among families living together at the time of the transmission would be helpful. Theoretical constructs speak mainly to reactions that family members may have in the presence of posttraumatic stress in the family system rather than focus on what the meaning of this experience is for the family members. As the field of knowledge increases and more theories emerge on secondary traumatic stress (STS), the question of how to prevent such transmission becomes the next logical step in this area of research. Specific questions such as how and why some family members experience STS while others in the same family, living in the same situation, do not develop such symptoms are critical to understand for military families. It is possible that some family members are more at risk for developing symptomatology based on variables such as: their age and/or stage of development at the time; their baseline temperament from birth; pre-existing traumatic stress or exposures to chronic trauma or child adversity; their previously developed coping strategies for managing stress that have proven effective and readily available to them; their place in the birth order among children in the family; a caring relative, teacher, or coach outside the system who is able to shift a child's attention and focus away from the family and offers hopefulness for healthy ways to adapt to the stressful situation; or there may be something else still to be discovered that is protective of those children who are lucky enough to not develop secondary traumatic stress in the presence of traumatic stress in their home environment.

Theories on the transmission of familial traumatic stress have linked the presence of ambiguous loss and boundary ambiguity that results from trauma to creating an environment where trauma is able to flourish. In situations where trauma is untreated, undisclosed, and not discussed in the family, and it remains that way in a chronic manner over time, traumatic roots are likely to grow in the system. Once traumatic roots take hold in a family system, they become a new added stressor that the family must manage (see Figure 7.2) as the environment takes on a toxic nature of attachment disruptions and broken trust in the world being a safe place. Individual family members can develop coping behaviors that are based in surviving the traumatic stress day-to-day rather than developing healthy ways of coping and goals that are directed toward the future. Many family members living with chronic traumatic stress will turn to substance use to alleviate

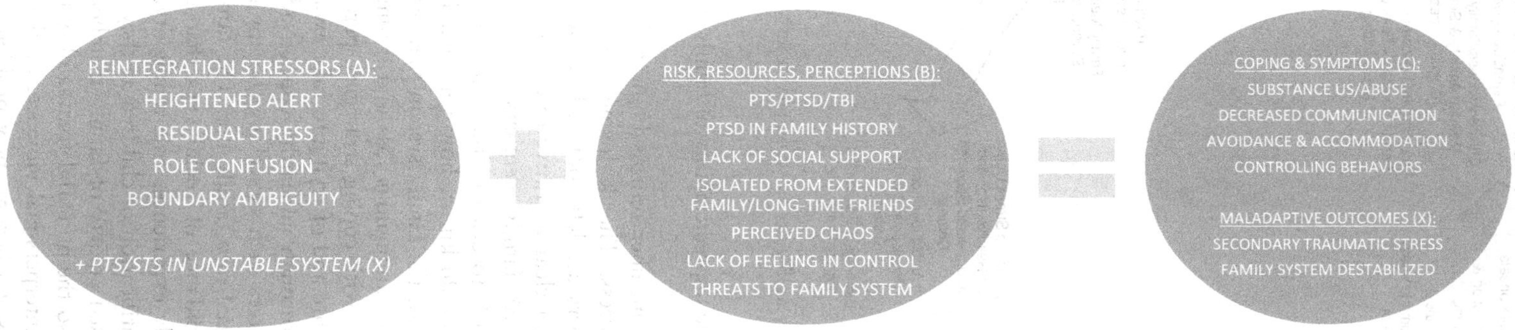

Figure 7.1 Interactional cycle of cascading effects in the family system with potential outcomes during reintegration phase following high-stress military deployment in at-risk families. (Potential effects illustrated through the lens of the Double ABCX Model of Family Adaptation to Stress of McCubbin & Patterson, 1983).

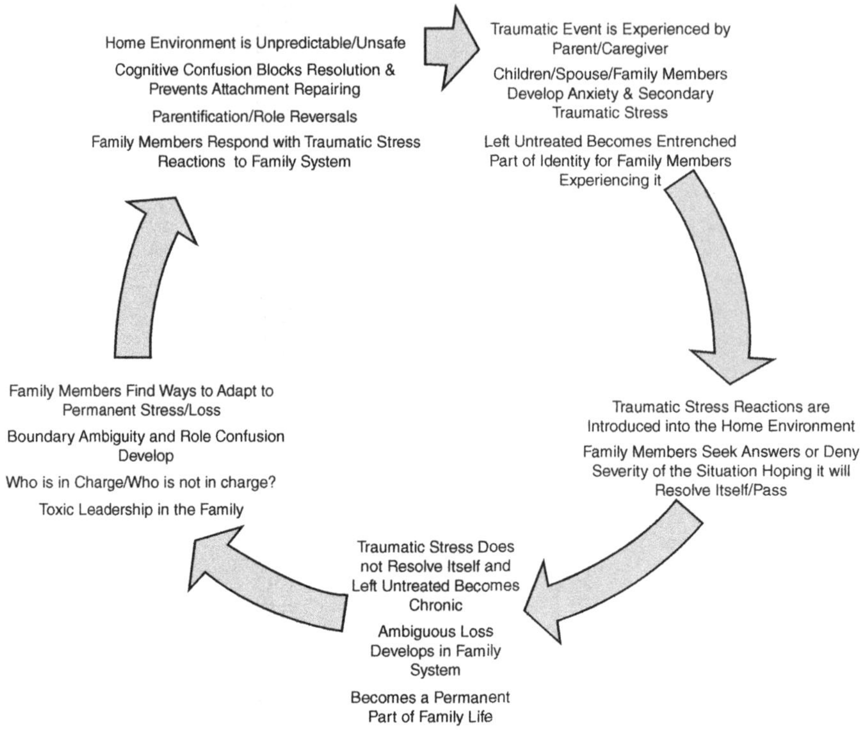

Figure 7.2 Role confusion and boundary ambiguity in secondary traumatic stress

the stress and attempt to manage the unpredictability of family life through numbing and avoidance techniques.

In Figure 7.2, a veteran service member returns home following a combat deployment with significant traumatic stress. The deployment is not discussed as being a traumatic event and family members are left confused about the changes within and between family members. Lacking a clear narrative to describe these changes, and the new family system that has emerged, family members cannot make sense out of this experience. The family has no words to describe the situation to themselves or to the world outside of their family. They do know, however, that family life has changed dramatically, and that they have lost the family system that was in place prior to the deployment. The family experiences ambiguous loss and traumatic stress reactions in daily life (A). The family responds with coping strategies, perceptions that the family will return to its previous way of life and of trying to take away the service member's stress (or denial of its existence through unhealthy coping, adaptations, and accommodations), and community resources such as seeking therapy in order to manage the daily stress that has been introduced into family life. The family attempts to accommodate to the stress through avoidance of social cues that trigger it and becomes isolated as a result (B). The family experiences role ambiguity, lack of clarity of leadership in the system, likely parentification of children as they assume both protective and limited parental roles, increased anxiety of family members, and secondary traumatic stress reactions. There is also the potential for inability to assume parental role requirements if substance abuse, interpersonal violence, or the risk for instability are present (C). All of these outcomes (C) become new problems for the family and the secondary traumatic stress becomes a way of life; the new daily way of coping is then a major risk factor to the family's ability to manage the stress, any future challenges, and their overall adaptive resiliency (X).

Family Accommodations to Posttraumatic Stress

Research with combat veterans and their families has established links between the presence of posttraumatic stress in family life and the psychological well-being of family members. According to a review of the literature, the numbing and arousal symptoms were reported to be the strongest influences on family distress and the addition of veterans' anger was associated with secondary traumatization among family members (Galovski & Lyons, 2004). In addition to this association, the majority of interventions with military-connected families have focused on reducing the veterans' symptoms rather than targeting the accommodations in the family system and the psychological well-being of the spouse and children. Veterans diagnosed with chronic PTSD were found to have more numerous and severe relationship problems, a higher divorce rate, and more difficulties overall in terms of overall family adjustment following military service. Male veterans with chronic PTSD were reported to be less self-disclosing, less emotionally expressive with their partners, and have greater anxiety related to intimacy following military deployments (Monson et al., 2009). The ambiguous loss that accompanies combat-related PTSD was reported to be problematic in one study as it led to role confusion among female spouses regarding whether the veteran was still functioning as a husband and independent adult or was now a dependent person in need of constant attention, much like having another child in the family (Dekel et al., 2005).

Role confusion and disrupted attachments from trauma in family systems require that treatments utilize a trauma lens and operate with trauma-informed care models for understanding familial behaviors and interactions. Traumatic stress reactions are anxiety reactions, based in fear, and sometimes displayed as anger or rage. When these occur in family life, there is an immediate response on the part of those family members not experiencing the reaction to take away the stress, and to alleviate the anxiety/fear/rage that is uncomfortable for everyone in the room. In attempting to do so, family members often make accommodations to distract others from it and to alleviate or prevent it from happening at the time and into future situations. Well-meaning family members will avoid situations that cause the reactions and in doing so, "accommodate the stress," which prevents it from getting resolved for the person experiencing the reaction. The posttraumatic stress will linger for as long as the family continues to make accommodations. The treatment consists of becoming competent at managing the triggers in the environment rather than avoiding them. In Figure 7.3, some of the ways in which traumatic stress is managed are described in terms of a primary parental figure having stress and the spouse/significant other accommodating to that stress by colluding with the social avoidance reaction. The family system becomes increasingly isolated over time as they decrease or stop attending social gatherings with friends, family, and in their community which poses a major risk factor for family resiliency.

The stages of trauma treatment include that safety and stability be established and maintained as the core components of any intervention that aims to understand behavioral communications and triggers of traumatic stress reactions. The differences between triggers that are found in the environment and triggers that are within an individual will be reviewed and understood as reminders of the traumatic event or situation that lead to great discomfort. The goals for such trauma treatment include distress tolerance, affect management, and to gain a renewed sense of competency in one's daily interactions in the world. Family members will often collude with denial or avoidance behaviors that result from traumatic stress

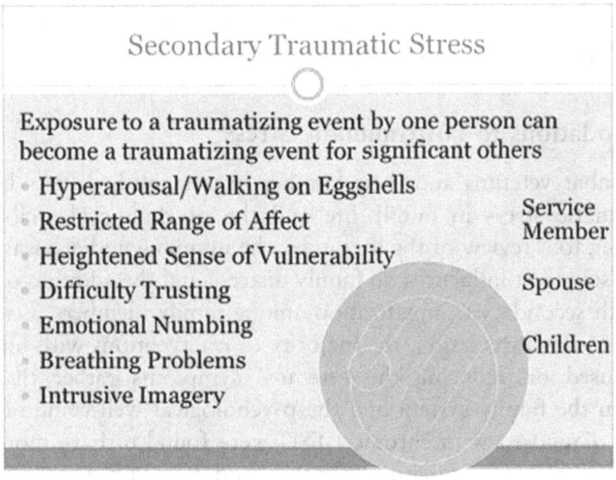

Figure 7.3 Secondary traumatic stress

reactions until such behavioral collusions are understood to be interfering with the goal of resolving the stress. The result of chronic over-accommodating of traumatic stress in families, through avoidance of its triggers, is reduced social engagement with extended formal and informal networks in the family's community. These include extended family, friends, significant partners, neighbors, coworkers, children's coaches, mentors, peers, and community overall at a time when social support is needed the most for resiliency. Helpful treatment includes interrupting the cycles of triggers and avoidance and are found in attachment-focused trauma treatments and emotionally-focused couples' therapy such as Sue Johnson's work with military couples (2019).

Environmental and Internal Triggers of Traumatic Stress

Some common examples of external triggers reported as related to military service include: sights and sounds, especially of fireworks; driving situations, particularly on highways or when other cars get too close; media and social media images related to war; children or adults who remind veterans of citizens of deployment countries or interpreters that assisted military missions; strong smells that remind someone of events such as barbecues and the smoke from a burning fire. Some examples of internal triggers include vivid recollections and/or dreams, thoughts, and memories of specific events, people, or places related to traumatic situations.

8 Injuries of War and the Military Family

Moral Injury in the Context of War

In 2021, the world saw the highly televised, media saturated withdrawal of U.S. military forces from Afghanistan. What media coverage didn't show, however, were the thousands of service members and veterans who had served in the war who watched at home, isolated from any military community. These individuals were unable to offer any support or assistance to the many interpreters who risked their lives for them who were texting, calling, and pleading for someone to rescue their families whose lives were at stake from their service to the U.S. military. The media did not show the sense of betrayal, guilt, and remorse experienced by so many veterans that day, left with the reality that the military machine had failed to do what many believed it should have done to keep those families safe. The military left them to cope with this reality on their own, without the social fabric of support they once had on active duty, in disbelief wondering about issues of morality, broken promises, and if there is ever a winner in war that takes so many lives on both sides.

Moral injury is the experience of having a deep sense of regret for failing to act in a manner that is consistent with one's values and morals, and in the context of war, this is generally an experience involving other human beings. Moral injury is an internal psychological process within an individual that is distinctly different from that of PTSD but often misdiagnosed as such in the current mental health field. The primary difference between the two is that moral injury is a psychological process and PTSD is a physical as well as psychological process and injury. The symptoms PTSD fall into the three clusters of intrusion, avoidance, and arousal and are internal psychological and physical reactions to triggers in the environment or within the individual followed by attempts to manage these reactions. The feelings of guilt, remorse, and shame may be present in both PTSD and moral injury and appear as overlapping symptoms from the same event, which makes the differential diagnosis difficult and complicated for many clinicians. The feelings from moral injury result from personal involvement in acts that have caused pain, suffering, and/or death, and are experienced across the realms of intellectual, emotional, and spiritual aspects of life. Moral injury can lead to significant changes in one's self-perception and often leads to depression, self-destructive tendencies, avoidance of positive experiences, and a general lack of hopefulness about the future. Morally injurious experiences are defined as events in which an individual perpetuates, fails to prevent, bears witness, or learns about acts that transgress deeply held moral beliefs and experiences which shatter moral and ethical expectations about fairness and the value of life (Litz et al., 2009).

In the context of war, moral injury arises from diverse causes including casualties to enemy combatants or civilians, giving an order that results in injury or death of service members, and witnessing the deaths of civilian casualties. Although the concept is not new, the term moral injury was coined in the mental health field following the era of

DOI: 10.4324/9781003438229-12

military service in Vietnam, as many veterans experienced a sense of betrayal of what is right by someone who holds legitimate authority, in a high-stakes situation (Shay 2002, 2010). Almost 40 years and several military involvements later, the concept continues to lack a formal diagnosis and the experience is not well understood by the majority of civilian mental health providers. Without a recognized diagnosis, mental health providers do not routinely ask about issues of morality or assess for this condition during sessions with veterans although all are well versed in the assessment of PTSD based on the diagnostic criteria for that condition.

In wartime, military service members often experience questions around issues of morality for participating in the horrific events that war entails. As one Marine combat veteran described it succinctly, "The military is a machine designed to do whatever it needs to do to accomplish its mission; it is a machine that will use its power for massive death and destruction and is designed to destroy anything that stands in its way." Service members who experience a sense of having violated their moral integrity often have great difficulty making sense out of this internally and integrating this aspect of their life into their identity. The challenge of how one explains this process to significant others such as close family members is often insurmountable, especially when one cannot explain it oneself. Due to this, mental health providers have an ethical responsibility to help their clients who experience moral injury to be able to find the words to describe, understand, and place this experience into a coherent narrative explanation. The lack of an explanation to understand one's experience in the world leaves the process unresolved and confusing for an individual who needs to answer the question of who they were before the event and how they have changed as a result.

PTSD refers to the mental and biological reactions that recur for months, and sometimes a lifelong struggle, that follows enduring or witnessing a traumatic event or series of events. The anxiety and fear that linger can bring about abrupt mood swings, avoidance of public settings, and withdrawal from social contacts. Individuals diagnosed with the disorder also experience hypervigilance, the state of extreme and heightened physical alertness that carries over from traumatic events. In some situations, feelings of guilt and shame can emerge months or years following a morally injurious event or series of events and linger in many negative ways. As service members adjust to the many layers of civilian life, the rationale for specific behaviors in war can loom as indefensible in hindsight, clashing with long-held personal beliefs, values, and perceptions of themselves, the military, and humanity.

Moral Injury Care and Treatment

Moral injury care has yet to be fully integrated into mental health treatments that are rooted in the medical model of diagnosis and treatment of symptoms as there is no place for issues of morality in a medical diagnosis. Moral injury lives in the realm of self-perception, calls for questions of redemption to be answered and involves finding a way toward resolving cognitive dissonance through cognitive and spiritual ways. In situations of interpersonal trauma, the act of forgiveness can be a goal of mental health treatment, either externally in reality with another person or as an internal process of forgiving another human being. Moral injury resulting from actively engaging in atrocities of war requires a very different kind of process, however, and often requires that acts of redemption take place in civilian life. This process may be one of several of the contributing factors that work together following military service that brings many veterans to works of charitable missions and altruism that can lead to healing, growth, and a renewed sense of self and self-perception as a morally intact person.

One mental health treatment for moral injury currently utilized is "adaptive disclosure" and the name speaks to the need for discussions of war-related issues that are adaptive in nature to cope with feelings that need resolution (Litz et al., 2016). As there is no formal diagnosis for moral injury, the majority of civilian mental health clinicians have not been educated or trained in initiating and holding such therapeutic discussions with military-connected individuals or families. The first step that needs to occur in such training would be for a civilian therapist to become aware of their personal preconceived biases and feelings held about the military and the acts involved in going to war. In the absence of such awareness, civilian therapists are not equipped to manage such discussions to be able to make them adaptive in nature, restorative, and healing. An obvious place to begin this therapeutic training is through curriculum studies in programs of higher education such as social work, nursing, and psychology focused on mental health treatment.

One part of adaptive disclosure treatment has the therapist guide a veteran through a conversation with a respected person, viewed by the veteran as a moral authority, to talk about the act or event that continues to haunt and impact that person's daily life. The client discloses feelings connected to specific acts of war that may include deep regret, and questions that person for ways to atone, similar to a religious or spiritual confession (Litz et al., 2016). As there is some degree of overlap between moral injury and spirituality, the care provided by chaplains working with veterans experiencing moral injury involves a collaborative approach, fostering trust, engaging in emotional processing and self-compassion, and working toward forgiveness and a future while living in the midst of suffering (Wortmann et al., 2022). The ability to tolerate painful feelings of guilt, remorse, self-condemnation and/or self-hatred while also holding the opposing view of positive hopefulness toward the future is often a very difficult process. The development of a trusting relationship with a therapist, clergy, or spiritual leader is often the cornerstone for moral injury care that is restorative and healing in nature. Without a positive therapeutic or working alliance for this process, the individual experiencing moral injury could employ maladaptive coping measures, resign him or herself to living with this being unresolved, and withdraw from the process entirely.

Moral Injury and the Military Family

Living with deep regret over violating one's moral compass, even when that violation was out of one's control during a military mission, complicates a return to daily living in the safe haven of family life. When veterans have difficulty accepting their personal involvement in wartime events, there may be a lost sense of pride in their military service and in themselves as a result. When one's identity shifts to incorporate a negative view of oneself, military service and/or civilian life can become complicated. One of the major aspects of depression includes cognitive shifts regarding one's beliefs about oneself, others, and the world and often distortions in these beliefs that have developed over time. Individuals who experience moral injury often carry with them a cognitive belief that what was once "all good" about themselves has become "all bad" with difficulty holding both self-perceptions simultaneously. This cognitive distortion is typical in the "all-or-nothing thinking" and is often a part of war where there are winners and losers and there is often life or death. Civilian family life is typically lived in the areas in between these polarized positions, however, and there are many shades of gray to navigate and tolerate. Parenting and family relationships are most fulfilling when there is at least some degree of joy and lightness that serves as a glue keeping bonds strong. Moral injury is devastating to intimate relationships for a myriad of reasons, from the overwhelming affective states of guilt and remorse over war-related experiences, to the toll it takes on daily functioning with cognitive confusion, self-doubt, and negative self-perceptions. It can easily feel impossible to believe that joy and remorse can coexist within a person's identity and psychological makeup as these often present as dialectically opposing affective states connected to opposing self-perceptions.

One recent study found that exposure to potentially morally injurious events among U.S. combat veterans involving transgressing or violating one's own core moral boundaries was associated with increased odds of lifetime alcohol and substance use disorders (Maguen et al., 2023). Exposure to such events that were caused or perpetuated by the individual were predominantly associated with alcohol use disorder while exposure that came from witnessing such events were predominantly associated with substance use disorders. The on-going presence of moral injury and persistent feelings of guilt and shame may lead to substance use to avoid and/or to numb difficult emotions. As the study concludes, similar to the ABCX model of adaptation to stress, harmful alcohol or substance use may result from perceptions of an inability to forgive oneself, self-condemnation, and/or self-loathing for failing to prevent acts that transgressed one's moral code. The substance abuse can also serve as a means of self-punishment, hopeless resignation, a cycle of functional impairment, and in the worst cases, can be fatal if it leads to a drug overdose or a completed suicide (Maguen et al., 2023). Research showing a potential link between moral injury, depression, and a higher risk of suicide highlights the risks and points to the need for mental health providers to introduce the topic for discussion in treatment sessions.

Military-Connected Injuries in the Family System

Veterans often describe the effects of living with PTSD as the metaphor of having a constant adrenaline drip that runs 24 hours a day and even when sleeping as this adrenaline interferes with getting a restful night of sleep. The switch for waking up and going to sleep that may have existed prior to a trauma often remains perpetually turned on and can remain that way for months, years, and even decades without treatment. The image of changing the on–off reactionary switch to one that has a dimmer on it is a useful tool for clinicians in helping to manage the effects of PTSD and place control back into the hands of the individual experiencing the effects. This imagery can also be useful as a stress-reduction strategy when sleep gets interrupted by nightmares or difficulty falling or staying asleep, particularly in combination with strategies for lowering physiological reactions such as heart rate or shallow breathing. The impact that sleep interruptions from traumatic stress can have on military family life is devastating as sleep is restorative and a key component of health and well-being. Traumatic sleep reactions can also impair intimate partner relationships if one partner in a couple sharing a bed is experiencing erratic sleep, physical stress reactions, or violent nightmares. Military spouses have adapted the saying "walking on eggshells" that typically describes daily living with someone with PTSD and added to it the term "sleeping on eggshells" following a deployment that was filled with trauma and stress. A partner who rolls over in their sleep may inadvertently cause a triggered stress reaction to occur in a veteran partner who is doing their best to contain an adrenaline response that is cued up for danger at any given moment in time. The damage that is caused by interactions such as these can include ongoing disruptions in sleep, threats to, or impairments in, the couple's attachment bond, physical and emotional intimacy problems, and risks to one's health and safety if a triggered reaction contains physical violence. Domestic violence advocates for partners of veterans and legal court advocates for veterans have debated the question of how to treat military couples in situations of intimate partner violence that is related to military-connected PTSD reactions. Some states and local jurisdictions have veteran courts that aim to divert veterans away from incarceration and into mental health treatment in the same states that prohibit mental health treatment for couples together when there is domestic violence.

The effectiveness of PTSD treatment is often influenced by certain risk factors that are associated with the military culture such as a general intolerance for mental health problems as these are viewed as potentially limiting the performance, safety, and stability of the military and its mission. There is an expectation among the military community that individuals and groups need to be strong and resilient in the face of adversity and seeking help can be seen as a sign of weakness or vulnerability which can prevent individuals from accessing treatments. In addition to the military context at large, other related and significant risk factors that discourage service members from openly discussing mental health concerns include: the internalized mental health stigma in military-connected communities; fears of being labeled mentally ill and perceived as dangerous; and the potential for negative career repercussions or discharge from military service as a result of being deemed unfit for duty in one's military occupational specialty. A complicating factor is also the frequent movement from one community to another, inherent in military life, that decreases the effectiveness of mental health treatments. Disruptions in treatments often occur when military families are required to relocate/PCS, leading to a forced and often premature termination with one's therapist and treatment team. The same happens when a military behavioral health provider is required to relocate and leave the therapeutic treatment prematurely, sometimes in the middle of a very difficult trauma treatment process, that can leave the military client at risk for deterioration across multiple levels of functioning. The need for coordination and collaboration among different treatment providers across state lines, sometimes with vastly different perspectives on mental health treatment, presents military clients and families with significant challenges to maintaining continuity of care that is beneficial to sustaining progress and achieving one's goals and/or positive outcomes.

Military families struggling with the effects of service-connected injuries and/or post-traumatic stress who have transitioned out of the military are at increased risk for experiencing social isolation and lack of social support in their new community networks. Since the nature of the military lifestyle requires frequent moves from one community to another, it is difficult to develop close relationships that are present in one's life for more than two to three years at a time. It is rare that military families will move at the same time to the same new location with established close friends in the military. This results in a lack of a cohesive social network that one might otherwise turn to in times of distress, as well as decreased awareness of social support programs available in civilian communities. The evidence presented underscores the critical role that having a sense of community support and sense of belonging plays in enhancing resiliency through PTSD programs. Research has consistently demonstrated that having a sense of community and social support are key factors in mitigating the negative impact of PTSD on military families and that this surpasses individual treatment or support (Franz et al., 2022; Bobrow et al., 2013). These studies also point to the importance of fostering a strong sense of community ties and networks of attachment that can facilitate healing and bolster resilience as a result. By prioritizing the development of supportive networks, creating opportunities and spaces for shared experiences, building new group identities, and increased belonging, such programs can significantly enhance the resiliency of military families living with PTSD. A community-based approach embraces the inherent strengths that exist within communities, harnesses the collective competence, and in doing so empowers individuals to be able to overcome adversity, ultimately leading to improved well-being and long-term resilience.

One study found that the greater the level of neighborhood cohesion, the lower the effect that PTSD had on parenting difficulties due to the positive effect of social connections and support networks (Franz et al., 2022). Multifamily therapy (MFT) has emerged as a highly effective and community-based treatment for PTSD in veterans (Van Ee et al., 2018). It offers unique advantages in addressing the negative impact of PTSD on their relationships and overall family functioning by placing families into a larger community of families sharing similar experiences that are distressing and thereby reducing the social isolation experienced by any one family. Studies have reported a correlation between PTSD symptoms and marital distress among veterans (Pflieger et al., 2022), highlighting the importance of implementing a treatment approach that emphasizes mental health and takes a familial perspective. MFT involves screening families by age of their children and screening for whether the military member has received what is referred to as "pre-treatment" prior to the sessions to prepare them for the possibility that they might experience traumatic triggers or overwhelming emotional reactions in the course of the treatment. Ideally, the military would lead such informational sessions for veterans in large group settings, in a military environment that would offer the safety of the familiar culture as well as the anonymity necessary to learn how to manage posttraumatic stress reactions without shame or stigma. If such groups were led by the military in a manner that normalized service-connected posttraumatic stress following discharge or retirement, veterans might feel ongoing support from the military and be less isolated in civilian life. The military has prevention programs (such as Battlemind in the Army and the Combat Operational Stress Continuum in the Marine Corps) that have been used to normalize and educate service members on certain behaviors that may have been adaptive for a military deployment but may be maladaptive in a civilian setting. Programs such as these are helpful in that they offer veterans a language for understanding and talking about behaviors that may be causing difficulties in their lives following military service. Resiliency programs that address social, emotional, and behavioral difficulties from an educational perspective offer alternatives to traditional mental health treatment that could prove helpful and be more accessible for veterans and military families.

Military Family Caregiving

The Veterans Health Administration has a program called "The Caregiver Program" and it is available to family members of veterans with a high disability rating, typically at 100%, as a result of their military service. This disability rating often includes the disability of PTSD, and sometimes PTSD on its own, and some researchers and providers have called into question the ethical implications that result from having a high disability rating solely for PTSD for two main reasons. The first reason is that being given a permanent disability rating for PTSD can potentially, and inadvertently, send the message that PTSD is a permanent disability that an individual must suffer with for the rest of their lives when this is not entirely accurate. There are many effective and evidence-based treatments for PTSD including trauma-focused cognitive behavioral therapy, cognitive processing therapy, and EMDR (eye movement desensitization and reprocessing) therapy. The current practice of assigning high disability ratings for PTSD is often referred to as the "lifetime disability rating for PTSD" as it tends to cause a disincentive to seek treatment and/or report improvements that could potentially decrease one's rating that is attached to income benefits. The second reason that lifetime ratings are seen as problematic is the military culture's emphasis on health, wellness, and strength that can leave a veteran with a lifetime of emotional pain, hopelessness for a more positive future, and social isolation as a result of accepting the condition as a permanent disability.

Suicide and the Military Family

Military organizations have recently begun to recognize the existence of previously misunderstood experiences of loneliness and social isolation among military-connected communities. The suicide rate of female Army soldiers while serving on a deployment was 3.1–3.5 times the rates of never-deployed or previously deployed female soldiers, while the rates for male soldiers on deployment was only 0.9–1.2 times the rates of other soldiers (Street et al., 2015). Some reasons that female service members may be more at risk for stress, depression, and suicide on deployments than their male counterparts include that there is significantly less social support for women on deployments since the majority of the military is male and deployment stressors may be mediated by social support, and the widely underreported prevalence of military sexual assault (the majority of which is perpetrated against women) that has been linked to suicide. In another study with 9,650 enlisted soldiers who had attempted suicide, 86.3% were male, 68.4% were younger than 30 years, 59.8% were non-Hispanic white, 76.5% had a high school level of education, and 54.7% were currently married (Ursano et al., 2016). The risk of suicide among enlisted soldiers who had never deployed was highest during their second month of military service. The risk for suicide among soldiers on their first deployment was highest during the sixth month of deployment. The risk among soldiers who had previously deployed was highest five months after they returned home. Soldiers who were on a deployment, or had previously deployed, were more likely to attempt suicide with a firearm than soldiers who had never deployed.

Given these statistics, suicide prevention efforts would include education and intervention efforts with specific military-connected populations. Female service members prior to leaving for a military deployment would be at risk for becoming suicidal on a deployment and because of this, detailed plans for safety would be beneficial as prevention measures. In addition to these safety plans, measures to increase social or health-related support during a deployment would prove helpful in some ways. Increased trainings on military sexual assault need to be in place prior to a deployment for all genders with plans clearly outlined for reporting to an outside source in the event of a sexual assault with a provider trained in confidentiality and reporting in the military justice system. Suicide prevention efforts would also benefit male service members (18–30 years old) with a high school level of education within the first month of military service, as well as during the first few months of a deployment, and within the first few months after returning home from a deployment.

Service members/veterans with deployment histories and their family members would benefit from prevention efforts that include education and information on the connection between having a history of a combat deployment and suicide by firearm. In addition to the service members being given the appropriate amount of education to increase their overall psychological well-being and fitness-for-duty, their spouses or significant family members (such as parents, siblings, or close friends of single or divorced soldiers) as well as any relevant care providers, should also be given this educational information so they can help to prepare for these situational crises to prevent them from happening and assist in times when prevention efforts have not increased stability and resiliency.

One report analyzed available research from international veteran communities on the similarities, differences, and reasons that military veterans are experiencing these constructs in current civilian communities and culture (Wilson et al., 2018). The authors describe loneliness as a subjective social and emotional experience that is characterized by the discrepancy between the social relationships we have and the social relationships we wish we had. Social isolation is an objective state that describes an individual in their social environment and includes the frequency of their social interactions and the presence or absence of social networks. Individuals can experience loneliness and social isolation together and these are often linked to poor physical health and well-being, including an increased risk of high blood pressure, cognitive decline, depression, and mortality. In the military context, social isolation has been demonstrated to increase the risk of marital distress, familial dysfunction, and suicide in military families (Wilson et al., 2018). In this review of studies on social isolation of military veterans, these authors reported that military service caused veterans to be uniquely vulnerable to the dangers of social isolation. The unique experiences found in military service, the presence of traumatic situations, and the multiple geographic transitions of military life contributed to an overall heightened risk of social isolation and its negative consequences on mental health and quality of life. This report linked the strain of social isolation inherent in the mobile military lifestyle, and the lack of support structures that are crucial for maintaining healthy relationships over time, to heightened stress levels, reduced coping skills, and decreased well-being.

Some common reasons reported for the transition out of military service being so difficult included the loss of the strong affiliative bonds between service members that create a family of individuals who care about and for one another. The literature highlights the intensity of friendship bonds formed during military service as providing one of the cornerstones of military identity and the practice of considering the military as one's family. In this perspective, military superiors (especially senior non-commissioned officers) fall into the role of a father figure and peers as brothers and sisters. Leaving military service results in these bonds being broken, with familiar and comforting family roles unable to fulfill these missing social bonds outside of the context of the military lifestyle in the context of the civilian world following military service. Loneliness and social isolation can easily lead to situations of despair without social support networks and treatment that is syntonic with the military culture. As military service members are trained on the use of weapons, these are often present in military family life as a source of protection, yet in the presence of serious declines in mental health, these pose the highest safety risks and need to be relocated to outside of the veteran's home.

In terms of help-seeking, one study found that male veterans (the majority of veterans), often delay posttraumatic stress treatment and are less likely to engage in help-seeking behaviors compared with female veterans due to traditional masculine ideologies that are perpetuated by the military culture and reported a desire to avoid thinking about and reliving traumatic events (Silvestrini & Chen, 2023). The majority of veteran suicides are by firearm weapons at the rate of 50% of female veterans and 70% of male veterans dying by self-inflicted gunshot wounds (U.S. Department of Veterans Affairs, 2021). Veterans are at increased risk for reaching the point of being suicidal including a cultural tolerance for lethality and the ever-present threat of death that is inherent in many aspects of military service. Several other risk factors are present including the loss of social support systems and networks in the military organization; the loss of identity of being a military service member, especially when difficulties transitioning to civilian roles are experienced; and the cultural stigma against help-seeking behaviors in the military. Combat veterans experiencing moral injury, unresolved posttraumatic stress, and chronic health conditions from service-connected injuries are at risk for adaptation to stress and resiliency if living without social support networks. According to the Veterans Health

Administration, there were approximately 17 veteran suicides per day reported in 2019 and the majority of these were with the use of lethal weapons. As stated previously, the use of firearms accounted for 70% of male veteran suicides in a slight increase from the previous year and almost 50% of female veteran suicides in an increase from 41% in the previous year. Veteran sub-populations reported to be at elevated risk for suicide included: female veterans, veterans aged 18–34, Native American veterans, Asian-American/Pacific Islander veterans, LGBTQ+ veterans; veterans with serious medical conditions; and aging veterans.

Despite the prevalence of veteran suicides in this country, there is scarce research regarding how suicide impacts the mental health of the family members left behind. The majority of veteran suicides occur in the home and are typically found by the veteran's spouse or children in the family. The term used to describe this experience is that of "suicide exposure," which means experiencing another's death by suicide. When this death is a significant family member, the resulting effects on family members is typically that of devastation, regret, guilt, self-blame, sadness, confusion, loss, anger at the military for causing and then not helping; anger at the civilian world for not helping or understanding the veteran experience … and trauma. One study conducted with National Guard troops describe PTSD and moral injury as separate constructs, with unique signs and symptoms, but the combination of PTSD and moral injury significantly increased the risk for suicidal thoughts and behaviors (Bryan et al., 2018). The concept of "suicide exposure" is discussed in the literature for the effects of a completed suicide on service members, veterans, and military families (Peterson et al., 2022). Data reported states that suicides overwhelmingly occur in the individual's residence (Defense Suicide Prevention Office, 2014). As a result of suicides occurring in the home, family members are the ones that are likely to find the body, which is an overwhelmingly traumatizing experience for these individuals (Harrington-LaMorie et al., 2018). Following a military death, the bereaved family members are required to undergo a military death investigation due to implications surrounding the deceased's benefits and life insurance policy; in addition to the grief and trauma, family members of a military suicide may experience greater shame, isolation, or distress than civilian families following a suicide (Harrington-LaMorie et al., 2018).

Suicide exposure among civilian populations has been reported to be associated with many negative outcomes, including feelings of rejection and shame, anxiety, depression, PTSD, complicated grief, as well as suicidal ideation and attempts (Peterson et al., 2022). Veterans, service members, and their families have unique challenges as a result of the military lifestyle including a history of attachment disruptions from deployments and long-term separation from their families-of-origin for active-duty families. These cultural factors can increase the risks following suicide exposure and result in prolonged grief as a result. A review of the literature reports that the rate of suicide exposure for veterans and military service members ranges from approximately 47% to 65% and the average for this population was reported as knowing three people who died by suicide (Peterson et al., 2022). These authors point out that given the high number of veterans and service members who know at least one person who died by suicide, the chances are high that family members of veterans and service members have also experienced alarmingly high rates of knowing someone who died in this way.

Family members of military service members who had died by suicide reported several areas that could be targeted for the prevention of military suicides including: reducing mental health stigma; increasing care and support from military leadership; providing confidential mental health and crisis intervention services; and increased awareness of the red flags or warning signs for suicide (LaCroix et al., 2018). The Defense Suicide Prevention Office identified several areas that raise risk levels for military service personnel as being related to the unique demands of the work and lifestyle known as "military-specific suicide risk factors." These risk factors include the following: demographics of the population drawn to military service; exposure to combat and high-stress environments being associated with higher rates of depression, anxiety, moral injury, and post-traumatic stress; the military culture that values toughness and discourages help-seeking behaviors; perceived stigma attached to mental health care, concerns that seeking care will harm their career opportunities; increased suicidal ideation, attempts, and death found among people with traumatic brain injuries; presence of increased risk of suicide among people who have substance use disorders, including heavy alcohol use, and a higher percentage of military personnel reporting heavy alcohol use compared to their civilian peers; having a loaded firearm in the home is reported to increase the risk for suicide by four to six times and service members are more likely to own a personal firearm than civilians (Kamareck et al., 2021). This report added that firearms are the most common method of suicide in military populations, accounting for 78.7% of suicides in the National Guard, 66.2% in the Reserves, and 59.6% in the Active Component in 2019. In terms of demographics, more than 90% of military suicides are men, and approximately half of reported suicides are junior enlisted personnel (E1–E4); while 42.7% of the total military population in 2019 were enlisted men under the age of 30, this demographic accounted for 61% of the reported suicide deaths.

There is a scarcity of research that has been conducted with families of veterans and military service personnel at this time although advocacy groups have called for more research, reporting, and collecting data on the experience as well as data on military spousal suicides and suicides of military children and children of veterans. This absence of research with military family members and friends of service members and veterans who have committed suicide point to the role that stigma continues to play in the military culture in addition to the huge sense of responsibility, shame, and guilt that is experienced as well. Given the high degree of distress following suicide exposure among military peers and family members, researchers have also called for strategies to be developed following suicides to decrease the risk of suicide contagion that has been documented (Hoge et al., 2017). The fact that suicide exposure among military-connected populations is a known and prevalent risk factor for future suicide points directly to the need for more qualitative research to understand the veteran and his or her military family experience. In addition to further research aimed at prevention, more research needs to focus on intervention strategies for the families left behind following a military-related suicide to manage the trauma and the crisis that presents itself.

Military Medical Retirements (Case Example)

In 2019, Army Staff Sargent Samuels discovered that while he was being trained on a new weapons qualification course designed to be more combat-oriented, with changing positions for urban combat situations, he began to experience memories and reminders of specific (traumatic) events from one of his deployments that he hadn't thought about in a very long time. These memories rendered him unable to reach his targets and maneuver at the same time on this new weapons training program. Although he tried on several occasions, he could not pass the necessary requirements of the new rifle marksmanship course that required him to engage targets faster and to operate as he did on a previous combat deployment. In a move to make Infantry soldiers more combat-ready, the trainings were very realistic by design, and this caused Staff Sgt. Samuels to become frozen every time he picked up a rifle. He told his commanding officer what was happening and why he was unable to pass his weapons qualification and was referred to medical command. The behavioral health officer at medical command recommended that he needed a profile limiting his duties and referred him to the Veterans Health Administration off the base for evaluation and counseling.

The Veterans Health Administration social worker determined that Staff Sgt. Samuels met the criteria for PTSD from military service and he was given a high disability rating based on his symptoms that caused him to be "unfit for duty" since his MOS was 11-B, an Infantry soldier. Staff Sgt. Samuels was shocked when he was informed of this as being an Infantry soldier was his entire military career and identity. Filled with shame and disbelief at the news, his self-perception changed drastically as he was about to lose his job and everything that was once familiar to him despite all his training and experience, because he was unable to control his emotions. Given his strong military cultural identity surrounding being a combat-arms soldier, he became depressed and unable to get out of bed, as he could not bear to be around his unit due to the sense of humiliation he experienced.

He was medically retired from active duty and moved into a civilian community with his spouse. Although he had attempted to form friendships with his civilian neighbors, these connections never became more than superficial and he experienced great sadness and isolation as a result. Staff Sgt. Samuels had lost his sense of identity, his community of peers who shared this cultural identity, and his sense of belonging. He began to have increased symptoms of posttraumatic stress, difficulty sleeping at night, and episodic rage directed at his spouse, the only person he interacted with on a daily basis, as he continued to grow more socially isolated over time. He did not need to get a job outside of the home since he received monthly disability income although he had heard of a program through the V.A. called Vocational Rehabilitation that he considered trying if he felt better sometime in the future. As he became more isolated, he became depressed and more dependent on his spouse, which caused him to perceive himself as a burden and to feel guilt and remorse for the entire situation. His spouse found out that they qualified for the Caregiver Program at the V.A. and was contacted by a social worker monthly who offered support services in addition to her being given a monthly stipend for not being able to work outside of the home due to taking care of him on a daily basis. Staff Sgt. Samuels became clinically depressed over time and expressed feelings that he would be "better off dead" to his spouse who would collect his life insurance and be freed from the burden of taking care of him.

His spouse called the social worker at the Caregiver Program and he was enrolled in a six-week residential program based on his symptoms of PTSD, depression, and heavy alcohol use that he was using as a daily coping strategy to manage his situational stress. Following discharge from the group residential program that offered him a sense of community, he returned home and received a therapy dog trained to wake him up from nightmares, divert his attention away from internal stress reactions, and to go into public places and be able to manage unpredictable environmental triggers of his PTSD. Once he was able to decrease his social isolation as a coping strategy, he was able to engage in outpatient trauma-focused therapy and his symptoms improved greatly over time. He applied for the V.A.'s Vocational Rehabilitation Program and attended college using his G.I. Bill benefits. He learned to transfer his skills of leadership, discipline, and physical fitness to a new profession and became a gym teacher and hockey coach at his local public high school.

9 Military Families Transition to Civilian Life

Military Families in Transition

In what is likely the most accurate and expressive title for a published research paper on this important topic, "Military Spouses Transition Too!" is a call-to-action paper that delves into the transition experience for military spouses separate from the veteran family member (Keeling et al., 2020). The military to civilian transition (MCT) experienced by military personnel as they discharge or retire from military service and enter civilian life is known for being challenging across a range of areas including employment, health, social supports, and integration to a new community. While military service members are offered multiple supports, trainings, and programs to assist them through the process of transitioning to civilian life, no such support exists for military spouses or children who have often been living with that same service member for the duration of their active-duty military career (Keeling et al., 2020). These authors report that in a review of research available, the needs of military spouses tend to focus on two areas: (1) the reintegration experience when the veteran returns to the family following a deployment; and (2) spouses who assume caregiving roles for mentally or physically disabled veterans in the post-deployment experience. Although there is limited research and knowledge about the needs of military spouses (and even less for military children), the issues that impact service members during the transition to civilian life also impact military spouses as well.

> *"My soldier retired from Active Duty 10 years ago. After 23 years of PCS'ing to 13 duty stations across the globe for anywhere from six months to six years, retirement seemed like a new, unexplored territory: staying in one place, putting down roots, starting a new chapter.*
>
> *Active Duty ended with a flurry of activity: retirement activities, out-processing, job hunting, house hunting, graduating a high school senior and transitioning to college. All in less than three months. When the dust settled and the movers dropped us off at our quarters— I mean our new home—I was unprepared for all the quiet.*
>
> *I had watched my husband prepare for his transition to civilian life, but never thought about my own. The quiet surrounding me was the absence of my "military family" family, that instant network of spouses and kids who filtered in and out of our lives for 23 years. I had to work to find some level of commonality with neighbors, and even speak a new language. Apparently, civilians do not speak in acronyms, shop at the PX and Commissary, and navigate around TDYs and deployments. This was not just a new chapter, but a whole new story, and one that needs time to unfold in this new, very quiet, very still, life we are living."*
>
> Military Spouse in Transition

DOI: 10.4324/9781003438229-13

In an effort to improve the transition experience for military spouses, successfully obtain desired employment, adjust to new civilian communities, maintain good physical and mental health, and achieve overall life satisfaction in their new civilian lives, military spouses were asked about their experiences (Keeling et al. (2020). Military transition theory (MTT) that had been developed previously to understand the service member's transition experience from military service to civilian life (Castro et al., 2015) was utilized as a guiding conceptual roadmap. Three of the significant constructs from MTT were applied to the military spouse's experience in the transition out of active-duty military life including approaching, managing, and assessing the transition to civilian life. Military spouses reported that they transitioned similarly with questions and concerns across the same areas as veterans including: education and employment; community, culture, and identity; marital relationships and family; health and well-being and had similar help-seeking behavior patterns as veterans (Keeling et al., 2020).

A review of the literature finds that military spouses (93% of whom are women) experience a "substantial and pervasive labor force penalty" for being married to someone serving in the U.S. military (Keeling et al., 2020). This labor force disadvantage is due to the reality that many, if not most, military spouses end up with work histories that are inconsistent with "the ideal worker" norms that are expected and valued by employers, such as a consistent employment in a consistent location. The strategies reported that military spouses use to adapt to this disadvantage, including taking part-time or volunteer positions, or furthering their education, often work against them as they have work histories of jobs that require less education or skills than they possess. Military spouses with higher education levels reported more perceptions of employer bias against military spouses; Army and Navy spouses were reported to earn a lower financial return on a bachelor's degree than civilians; and all military spouses earned a lower return on a graduate degree than did civilians. Following chronic periods of unemployment, underemployment, and perceived employer bias, some military spouses were reported to have lowered or abandoned their career aspirations altogether and opted out of public labor force employment and into roles of volunteering or family caregiving (Keeling et al., 2020).

Many military couples struggle to rebuild a social network of friendships, neighborhood acquaintances, and social connections in one civilian community following the transition out of active-duty military service. In addition to this struggle, many military couples report challenges in re-creating intimacy, conflict resolution in their relationship, and establishing new identities in relation to one another and with their families-of-origin. Couples also reported challenges in shared decision-making and re-establishing safety and trust in the relationship; these areas require effective communication skills which were often compromised due to lengthy separations, role shifts, and long stretches of time apart in the military (Keeling et al., 2020). Additionally reported were that dual-military couples may experience heightened challenges during the transition process especially if psychological injuries from trauma or moral injury were experienced by both partners, as this could also influence couple and parenting abilities. The overwhelming majority of research concerning the veteran's experience has left out the subjective experiences of the military spouse and children. Many psychotherapy treatments for marital conflicts with veterans tend to focus on reduction of the veteran's symptoms with little to no consideration of the military spouse's intersubjective experience as an equal participant in the situation.

In addition to the areas of employment and overall well-being, military spouses have also reported anecdotally having difficulties adjusting to civilian life across the domains of internal experiences in areas that include their relationship with their partner, establishing civilian friendships, and remaining located in one geographic location or dwelling for the rest of their lives. The experience of living an active-duty military lifestyle for up to 20 years for many couples results in certain habits that are formed as a result. These habits include daily living that has been characterized by years of sacrificing their own needs and wants for the military and the service member's career in the military. Spousal needs have never taken priority because the military mission always came first throughout the couple's time on active duty and the service member's career that was attached to those military missions. Military spouses have reported a significant shift when the family transitions out of military service following the move to the new location to start the next phase in family life in a civilian community. Military support systems and networks are in place on active-duty bases and finding acquaintances or even short-term daily friendships is never too difficult if these are desired. These may not be sought out in times that families want privacy, however, as living in close proximity can be stifling when one's private life is relatively public information such as often occurs in active-duty military communities. The supply, availability, and opportunities to develop social relationships on active-duty bases is present if a family member wants to engage socially with one's neighbors and community. Finding and developing social relationships in civilian communities is often much more difficult to establish as the formal support structures are not the same and may not exist at all in certain neighborhoods. In addition to the lack of social structures in place that present opportunities to develop social relationships, civilian communities may have a sense of neighborhood cohesion already established. Military service members who may be single, never married, or divorced and military families who have been on active duty for 20 years often move into neighborhoods where civilian families have lived their entire lives and have long histories with one another.

Civilian children have often attended the same schools as their neighbors, celebrated holidays together, played on the same sports teams, joined clubs, summer camps, and after-school activities together in addition to accumulating memories from daily life events too many to mention. The permanence that is often a hallmark of civilian life can present very challenging obstacles for military families to navigate to establish new friendships, new relationship bonds, and to build a completely new social support network. In addition to the situational challenges of building such a support network, military family members may not possess the skills necessary to create social networks without the infrastructure that was present and familiar in military communities. The initial period of time following the transition out of the military into civilian life is a critical one in terms of mental health and overall well-being for military families. Military spouses often report feelings of loneliness, isolation, confusion about roles, identity, unsure of how to overcome these challenges, and are at heightened risk for depression at this time as a result. Military children are equally at risk due to the same reasons and moving into neighborhoods and schools with groups of children who have grown up together, negotiated conflicts over time, discovered their peer groups, and settled into the tasks of growing up. In addition to the challenges found with integrating into new civilian social groups, military children often report anxiety associated with school especially if they have academic learning difficulties or neurodiversity in their learning styles. Military children may also experience social challenges as they adjust to relationships with their civilian peers who may not be familiar with the military culture, behavioral expectations, and/or the collectivist perspective.

Since the family has moved every two to three years, the notion of settling down in one place may be romanticized over time when moving difficulties arise, yet the permanence of not moving again is often a difficult adjustment for family members to make. Moving becomes part of the family's identity. The experience of being highly mobile and ready to pack one's entire life at any given time becomes an ingrained part of family life.

Oftentimes around the point of a few years following the transition to a civilian neighborhood, some military service members and their spouses report wanting to move again, and many will identify the geographic location outside the military installation where they experienced the most life satisfaction. Many young adult military children will move with their parents as the concept of the family home is wherever the parents move next rather than in a geographic location. Childhoods marked by multiple geographic homes lead military children who grow up on active duty to have difficulty answering the question "Where are you from?" The answer to this common question is often simply "Everywhere and nowhere."

If the couple has children in the family, the children likely came next in terms of needs given their ages and dependency needs. As the family has typically moved every two to three years, the focus on relocating took priority as well since a geographic move of a family requires significant planning and logistical operations often done by the military spouse. In unpaid labor, a military spouse begins planning a family move immediately upon getting notification orders of where that move may, or will be, in terms of investigating housing and school situations at the new location. This process usually begins not long after the previous move has happened and the family has finally settled into the location where they are at the time. Community resources need to be located and appointments scheduled before a move for any specialty healthcare and more recently generalized dependent healthcare in some locations has been transitioning off active-duty bases and into the civilian community. Many community providers do not have contracts to work with Tricare/Humana, the military insurance company that manages healthcare for military families, and "out-of-network" referrals need to be approved/secured by the case manager on the base for many community providers. If any family members need specialty services such as physical therapy, occupational therapy, mental health therapy, orthodontic needs, academic testing, psychiatric medication management, and many others, community providers off base need to be found and figuring out payment for these services needs to be negotiated between the family and the insurance company. This work typically falls on the active-duty spouse to research, manage, and often advocate for services to begin as soon as possible if there are very long waiting lists in the community. In terms of mental health treatment, therapy with providers is interrupted/terminated with every move and military families need to start the process of finding new behavioral health providers licensed in the new state. The recent pandemic lifted restrictions (such as getting prior authorizations and responsibility for co-payments) and ushered in a period of telehealth that took the burden of getting to appointments off base and negotiating with providers often much easier, especially for children. The majority of children, however, reported not feeling comfortable with telehealth for mental health treatment, and many made better progress with in-person therapies due to their developmental stages and lack of privacy using telehealth at home. Providers also reported less effectiveness in terms of not being able to see a client's body or read body language with telehealth that only shows a client from the neck up. Social workers and other mental health professionals who work with adolescents reported not being able to see if a teenager had certain issues with telehealth. Conditions such as an eating disorder of restricted caloric intake is usually evident in person and not with telehealth. Another adolescent behavior that that needs in-person therapy is the behavioral coping strategy of self-harm, that many teens engage in as a way to manage strong emotions when they do not have the necessary skills to do so. In assessing adolescent mental health, providers have a list of questions they ask as part of a clinical evaluation that need to be asked in confidential spaces as teenagers do not wish to upset their parents with their answers.

Adolescents in military families are especially sensitive to the concept of not upsetting their parents as they live in parent-focused families and because of this, in-person sessions are the most helpful. In addition to the list of questions regarding their histories and levels of functioning, two questions are particularly important to weave into assessments with military teens. The first question is simply: "Do you like school and reading?" to assess for potential reading disabilities and academic achievement toward reading goals for military teenagers who often have had six to seven moves in their lifetimes and enrolled in five to six different schools. As each school move may have been associated with academic losses and difficulties with developing social skills, this question offers valuable clinical information. If the military continues the practice of moving families as often as every two to three years, some advocates call for a federal school system for military youth. In previous eras, military families moved much less frequently, sometimes every four to six years, and military children sacrificed less in terms of their educational success, academic achievements, and associated mental health from decreases in these areas.

Another question that clinicians working with military teens who have transitioned to the civilian community following military service often ask as part of their ongoing work concerns feelings about the military lifestyle: "Do you want to be in the military yourself or start your own military family someday?" The military continues to uphold traditional gender-based stereotypes, and military youth who may be lesbian, gay, bisexual, transgender, or questioning their identities may not be able to do so openly or safely in their military communities but may feel more comfortable doing so following the transition to civilian life. They may also receive harsh messages and hateful speech or reactions when these topics are discussed in the home and across military-connected communities. For this reason, military teens need to have safe spaces where any topic can be explored with complete confidentiality. Topics need to be introduced with sensitivity in a non-judgmental manner as many military teens have spent their entire lifetimes assessing adults for what they can and cannot discuss and what consequences might arise for them as a result of any given discussion. The fact that military youth live in parent-focused families with gendered stereotypes that adhere to strict guidelines for behavior, explains why in-person mental health sessions are more effective than telehealth sessions for these youth. Military teens may prefer to use gender-neutral pronouns and this may not be acceptable in their families, but the use of the correct pronouns needs to be included throughout every treatment session. Military teens who may be experiencing racism, bullying, micro-aggressions or other forms of discrimination may be reluctant to open up such discussions out of concerns of raising anxiety levels for their parents but need to explore these topics in depth for their mental health, well-being, and to make plans for resolving problematic situations with a trusted adult.

In the transition to civilian life outside of the military, some of the previously adaptive coping strategies that had been useful in managing stressful situations and conflicts may no longer be adaptive or necessary following military service. Coping skills that may have developed in response to repeated and lengthy separations may involve a tendency to perceive relationship separations as restorative and healthy rather than representing loss or attached to any negative implications as a result. The shift to having all family members together at all times can be unique and challenging for some military couples and families who may have managed relationship conflicts best through separations and time spent apart. Although many military families work well as a team conceptually, doing so effectively may have always included time spent independently due to military work away from home and coordinating lifestyle demands. If family separations were helpful and adaptive in managing stress levels, this may present as a challenging adjustment for military families to make post-military service. The ongoing presence (up to 20 years for some families) of having a reprieve from family and social conflicts through physical separations leaves many families adapting to civilian life without one of their primary coping strategies. As civilian life does not need to have repeated interruptions in relationship attachments, conflicts in these attachment bonds may present as challenging for military family members who may need to develop different coping skills for conflict resolution in family and social relationships. As part of the transition from military to civilian life, families often need to create new family roles, new task responsibilities, and new collaborative problem-solving methods when stressful situations arise.

Issues surround the transition out of the military include the very personal meanings that are experienced and processed independently by the service member, spouse, and military children including the loss of community, shared purpose, and group and individual identity. Many service members hold an identity as a warrior first and foremost and the loss of this identity is significant for them and it is crucial to fully understand this psychological transition. In addition to this loss of individual personal identity, there is also a loss of the identity as being part of a group that works together at all times. The loss of a sense of group cohesion and connections with other warriors is often not given the level of importance that it deserves in terms of transitioning out of the military. Although the military has countless traditions and rituals for indoctrination into the system, it ignores this phase and process for leaving and most military service members leave the group to function in a civilian world that does not share the same values or collectivist mentality that has guided their lives and shaped their behaviors for many years. The loss of what is known as the "esprit de corps" is not just the loss of a group of people, it is the loss of identity, a way of being in the world, and for seeing the world, and all the issues that are related to the military perspective and way of life.

The Veterans Health Administration and Disability Ratings

Military members go through regular annual health assessments as routine parts of service to ensure fitness for duty across multiple areas of health and mental health that evaluate changes in areas that limit occupational abilities and functioning. When there is a change to a military service member's health, or fitness level for any reason, steps to return to previous levels and optimal health are required. Information concerning physical or mental limitations are documented on that member's "profile" of his or her fitness and ability to perform their role in their occupational specialty. These conditions can be temporary, such as a broken arm or a pregnancy, or they can be permanent such as a life-threatening illness or severe condition that is chronic and unresponsive to treatment. Military service members can sustain multiple physical injuries while on military duty including traumatic brain injuries, spinal cord injuries, injuries to motor skills, tinnitus, chronic migraine headaches, hearing or vision loss, and lung conditions from exposure to airborne hazards such as open burn pit smoke, oil well fires, and/or other pollutants. Service members may also experience psychological injuries such as posttraumatic stress, anxiety, depression, attention deficit disorders, and cognitive impairments that are included in one's profile for fitness for duty as well. The impact of an injury on one's occupational functioning is coordinated with the military medical command and the service member's unit command for that member's fitness for duty. When injuries exist that are a result of military service, these are "service-connected injuries" and in situations where injuries that limit occupational functioning are chronic, severe, and unlikely to improve, the military service member will go through a medical review board process and typically be medically retired from service. In military medical retirements that render a service member "unfit for duty" due to military service, that individual will be eligible to receive financial retirement compensation and healthcare benefits for the rest of his or her life for the permanent disability. This is disability income to compensate the service member for the limited future functioning and as such is not typically considered a marital asset should a military couple get divorced. The states all have interpretations of military divorce policies, however, and multiple complex algorithms have been discussed that encourage individuals to seek local legal counsel on these matters.

The Veterans Health Administration (VHA) in the United States is the largest employer of social workers in the United States and employs medical professionals from all medical disciplines including doctors, nurses, psychologists, psychiatrists, and other licensed mental health-care providers. Although this is changing across disciplines, many providers are not required to take military-specific courses as part of their academic training, and enter into this work with limited understanding of the military lifestyle. Providers learn about the culture through trainings offered through the VHA and the day-to-day working environment and culture present at most facilities. Veterans will often have multiple providers and social workers due to internships and training programs and may not be able to establish the same long-term therapeutic relationships available in the private sector of civilian life. Some veterans have reported that many of the case managers they work with do not make or maintain eye contact with them during their meetings or in treatment sessions. There is an irony in the fact that the majority of treatment providers at the VHA are social workers whose chosen profession is often opposed to the culture of patriarchy, hierarchical thinking, and the use of aggression that is reminiscent of the military culture. This cultural imbalance is rarely discussed in professional social work curriculum across both required and elective courses yet has an effect on the relationships that are crucial to the therapeutic healing process with military-connected populations. The cultural competency training that is required for most health-care providers as part of their state licensing boards is often lacking topics on military culture despite the shared traditions, rituals, language, and customs that influence daily life. The ability to maintain eye contact in mental health treatment is a communication about trust and the overall safety of the treatment situation itself. The issue of trust is especially significant for veterans due to the nature of the military culture, the military training in situational awareness, and the role that trust plays in daily life following traumatic situations such as the experience of going to war.

Mental health treatment sessions often contain highly personal questions about traumatic experiences asked by providers who are required to enter responses as data into a computer. Some veterans have reported feeling disrespected by this process that is supposed to honor their military service and that the high rates of depression may even decrease with a more thoughtful approach to developing treatments that address the issue of trust. One of the most crucial parts of therapeutic healing lies in the creation of a strong therapeutic alliance based in trust that repairs feelings of isolation. Mental health treatment providers form positive working alliances and social connections with their clients through a professional code of conduct and ethical interventions in the process of healing. The chronic and heavy relational wounds that can follow wartime service cannot be resolved without bearing significant witness to the pain, suffering, and moral injury that may be present and require full and often painfully difficult relational engagement in the therapeutic process that follows such service.

Resiliency through Clinical Education and Policy Change

During the height of the post-9/11 wars, social work educators began to develop curriculum content for their students that focused on military and veteran issues to educate and raise the clinical competency levels in the profession. Since the VHA is the largest employer of social workers in the United States, this profession bears the responsibility for treating the mental health and well-being of veteran and military-connected communities. Spouses of veterans may participate in couples' counseling and receive supportive services focused around their veteran spouse at some VHA facilities and Vet Centers (that are part of the VHA yet keep separate records, policies, and procedures). The Vet Centers developed in the 1970s when many veterans had reported having negative experiences at the VHA and lacked trust in certain government policies and programs following the era of conscription into military service in Vietnam. The Vet Centers are available to combat veterans only and many staff are combat veterans themselves or military-connected family members. Military spouses and children of veterans are not eligible for therapy without the veteran being involved in that treatment at the VHA or the Vet Centers. The question of "why not?" has yet to be brought up in political arenas as active-duty military spouses and children are eligible for mental health treatments on bases and when referred to community providers. This can be problematic in cases that involve interpersonal family violence between the couple and/or a spouse managing a family system with a veteran who is severely depressed and at risk for suicide. Both of these life-threatening situations often require anonymity in mental health treatment, which is not possible with current policies in place through these facilities, yet could open up many avenues for improving the situation. The situation of a child or family member finding their loved one dead by suicide, most often by a gunshot wound to the head, could possibly be prevented from happening with thoughtful shifts in policy around family-based therapeutic interventions for veteran and family well-being.

The issues of whether this system bears the responsibility for treatment for military spouses and children of veterans on their own accord, with or without the presence or consent of the veteran family member, is largely invisible in current social policy debates. Military-connected families deserve quality mental health treatment funded by the federal government through VHA programs. As the Vet Centers emerged following military service in Vietnam, the current era of the "all-volunteer force" has created a generation of veterans who served in the military while starting families and raised hundreds of thousands of children who have needs of their own as a result. At present time, there is no mental health treatment offered to spouses or children of military veterans. Military family and veteran treatment centers have developed with funding from private philanthropy and often located in large urban settings. While these offer excellent alternatives to civilian mental health providers for veteran families, there are too few of these and far between, not accessible to all families such as those living in rural settings, and without guarantee that private philanthropy will always be available. These treatment services would benefit from federal funding streams to ensure their sustainability for future generations of military families to thrive and to address child maltreatment, family violence, secondary traumatic stress, marital dissolution, and veteran suicides.

Following the first decade of war post-9/11, the social work community of educators began to hold an annual "Military Social Work" conference to provide opportunities for educators, clinicians, researchers, and thought leaders to come together for information-sharing, support, education, and insights into the volume of issues that were emerging in response to the wars. This conference continues with a very different approach and the sense of urgency at the time grew much quieter over the course of the second decade as the wars ended and many veterans transitioned out of military service, many medically retired from service-connected injuries. As the military is now recruiting its new generation of military service members from local high schools and outreach to the young adult populations, this next wave of military families is just beginning with babies being born to service members and families being established. As events in the political landscape threaten new conflicts around the globe, the military will once again call young service men and women to wartime military deployments and the new families will experience the cycle of deployment stress all over again.

As courses began to appear in schools of social work and other disciplines in response to the wars in Iraq and Afghanistan, some educators advocated for more focused curriculum content but there was a lack of agreement on the topic. According to some educators, administrations offered to support content on helping veterans, but not on the military, due to ethical and philosophical reasons. Although many schools of social work and other helping professions have established courses related to veteran issues, these courses are rarely required curriculum in any concentration and the students who elect to take these courses are more often than not student veterans and military-connected family members. If these courses continue as elective curriculum, there remains the risk that the content would become too specialized over time and remain self-selected by veterans and military-connected students.

After a decade of writing and teaching about military culture, veteran mental health, and transitioning to civilian life, researchers conducted a study to determine if these courses were improving clinical efficacy for students (Coll et al., 2012). The study explored military cultural competence in social work education, clinician self-efficacy, and its relationship to the participant's military experience and military-related coursework. The majority of students surveyed (70%) had experience working with veterans and 30% had completed at least one or more continuing education courses in military social work. The students who were veterans and military spouses reported higher levels of self-efficacy than did non-military students and results suggested that social work educators were "preaching to the choir" and that there was a need to integrate the content into the generalist curriculum. Topics including military social work, military culture, military/veteran behavioral health, and military family systems need to be included in mainstream social work education curriculum in the areas of diversity, aging, research methods, family systems and family therapy; macro policy courses; and Human Behavior and the Social Environment (Coll et al., 2012).

Despite the evident need for increased military-focused content to be included in social work education, from informal surveys from schools of social work, there is little content in many social work curricula concerning the effect of the military lifestyle, the culture, and the unique experiences of veterans and military-connected families (Canfield & Weiss, 2015). Most of the content that is delivered in social work education (if any content on service members or veterans and their families is provided) tends to link veterans with PTSD, its effects on daily functioning, and clinical psychotherapy treatment. Although this is a significant issue for the veteran population, it is one piece of a larger spectrum of potential outcomes that may affect military service members and their families. Issues such as anxiety, depression, substance abuse, and family stress are among the challenges reported by active-duty military personnel. The problem with this limited educational emphasis that is trauma-focused stereotypes the population incorrectly and does not fully equip a social work student with the broader sense of the experience of military culture and lifestyle. The unique culture of the military family and the veteran nested within that family is a very interesting, rich, and complex one that civilian social workers would benefit greatly from understanding. There are highly nuanced case studies and research with the military and veteran population that provide great insights into human behavior and the social environment, the intersection of race, class, culture, and the variety of social identity markers of cultures within military-connected communities, as well as provide opportunities for critical analysis in the areas of social work policy, practice, and research.

Student Veterans in Higher Education

More than 2.5 million post-9/11 veterans have returned from the wars in Iraq and Afghanistan and many have been pursuing higher education utilizing benefits provided by the U.S. government. Returning veterans are seeking to develop meaningful post-military service careers and financial stability, yet evidence suggests that student veterans are at risk in terms of being able to achieve academic success when compared to their non-veteran peers. While student veterans earn postsecondary degrees and certificates at rates similar to non-veteran students, time to completion is longer (Riegel, 2013). The slower completion rate is troubling because of the restrictions associated with the G.I. Bill that may not provide sufficient time for them to finish programs before their benefits are exhausted. Thus, student veterans often need to find alternative financial resources to complete their educational goals and this issue could result in their experiencing financial crisis, family disruptions, food and housing insecurity, and a host of related problems. Student veterans need to receive the appropriate amount or type of academic supports and accommodations necessary to complete their educational goals in a timely manner. Although there are a variety of support services as well as veteran spaces to address their needs, the efficacy of these programs remain largely unknown. Many institutions of higher learning identify as "military friendly," which projects a welcoming environment for student veterans, and some institutions of higher education have translated this concept into day-to-day practices such as matching certain benefits for cost-free education across campuses.

Transitioning out of the military also often means finding a new career in the civilian sector and this process comes with many risk factors as skills learned in the military are often not translatable to other careers and status that has been well-earned is no longer a part of their work life. Military service members are identified as veterans when they transition out of military service and this identity is often a difficult one due to significant stigma associated with this identity perpetuated by the media and generalized by many civilians as a result. Student veterans are enrolling in higher education with the assistance of the G.I. Bill and Yellow Ribbon Programs for tuition reductions and tuition-free if their G.I. Bill benefits are at 100% and the school has a policy for matching these funds. Student veterans with service-connected disabilities may present with the need for accommodations in the classroom and in their overall academic learning in higher education as a result of military-specific experiences. There are many physical accommodations that may be needed such as handicapped access to classrooms and student housing that may be single occupancy, on a first floor, or in a building with an elevator. Student veterans with long-term symptoms from concussions such as chronic fatigue and other ongoing health conditions may require academic accommodations including the following: extended time on tests and assignments; having a note taker for classes; the ability to use talk-to-text software or devices for writing lengthy papers; access to text-to-talk audio recordings for textbooks; testing in a separate and quiet location, with low lighting if the student has migraine headaches or tinnitus, and the ability to take frequent breaks and leave the room if necessary; priority registration for courses; part-time course load counted as full-time to not lose their student benefits; being allowed extra absences from classes during flare-ups of chronic medical conditions; having a service or trained therapy dog in classes, public spaces, and living in student housing to manage triggers of traumatic stress in the campus community. Many student veterans and military-connected employees do not wish to identify with their veteran status or connection to the military upon embarking on their careers for a host of diverse reasons. These reasons include a perceived stigma and stereotypes held by many civilians, together with the limited research on the experiences of student veterans as well as the intersectionality of being a veteran from a racial or ethnic minority. This intersection can lead students from underrepresented racial or ethnic minorities to experience heightened stress levels in classrooms and across college campuses and struggle to find welcoming spaces to voice their experiences and perspectives.

Racial/Ethnic Minority Student Veterans

College students need adaptive coping skills to be able to manage all the demands of academic life and this becomes more difficult if they experience any level of race-based hostility in higher education classrooms or public spaces on campus. Studies have reported that Black and Latinx college students are at heightened risk for depression and stress in response to racial/ethnic microaggressions, and this risk is elevated for those who attend predominantly White institutions (PWI) with limited institutional support (Hope et al., 2018). These microaggressions were reported as being common experiences for Black and Latinx students and perceived racial discrimination was associated with a greater prevalence of trait anxiety among Asian and Latinx college students (Hwang & Goto, 2008). The intersection of identity markers for student veterans of racial/ethnic minority backgrounds places these students at high risk for vulnerability in terms of feeling safe to learn fully and express opinions freely. Feelings of social isolation from underrepresentation on campus, greater stigma, and heightened levels of stress and anxiety have been reported as well.

Racial/ethnic minority students at PWIs have reported significantly more depressive symptoms and distress than White students. Two concerning themes were reported in one study on the experiences of Black male students enrolled in a PWI that included the experience of being stereotyped in terms of what others thought about them and their upbringing, and that Whites behaved extremely cautious and alert when they were around Black students (Smith et al., 2007). Many different coping strategies are employed by racial/ethnic minority students in racially hostile campus environments, and socio-political activism is one of these, in taking action through resistance to the experience of discrimination. It is not always adaptive across racial/ethnic minority groups, however, and one study found that while it improved anxiety for Latinx students, it worsened the overall mental health and wellness for Black students at the same PWI (Hope et al., 2018). Students who express concern about racial stigma in their institutions are more likely to experience negative mental health and have lower grade point averages than students who are less concerned about racial stigma (Brown & Lee, 2005). In addition to these issues, one study reported the great difficulty evidenced by graduation rates as only 40% of Black and 52% of Latinx college students obtain a bachelor's degree within six years of their initial enrollment (Snyder & Dillow, 2015). These concerning reports and figures reinforce the need for collective responses on the parts of predominantly White institutions of higher education to reduce discrimination, racism, and stigma and to foster non-hostile learning environments that are free from prejudice.

Challenges for Veterans in Civilian Life

Issues of post-deployment stress are routinely normalized within the military and referred to simply as "posttraumatic stress" without the disorder attached to the label. The life-changing nature of stress from serving in the military during wartime is often mistaken by civilians for the very debilitating condition of "PTSD" when in fact the disorder accounts for less than 20% of veterans from the last two decades of war. Civilian peers and employers who do not understand the military culture or perspective can easily misinterpret situations in negative ways if taken solely from the civilian point of view. There is a scarcity of information available to civilian employers in the current era to bring awareness to these experiences that are so multilayered in complexity that they are often misunderstood due to this lack of knowledge. As with any lived experience, the divide is often best bridged through honest and open communication on both sides, however only if that practice is welcomed and accepted.

Challenges faced following the military are many and often stem from the lack of strong social support networks that are crucial to military service members, their spouses, and their families. In addition to this significant challenge, many veterans also struggle with chronic pain from injuries in military service that can lead to chronic substance misuse, addictions, and depression. The loss of a sense of purpose without the military leaves many veterans facing difficulty transitioning into the civilian world as well as unexpected responses from civilians to behaviors that were normative within the military. The loss of support networks and a sense of purpose can lead to a loss of optimism, isolation, and at worst, thoughts of suicide perceived to be a warrior's death. Marital problems, family dissolution, financial worries, housing insecurity, and the persistent desire to return to military service all combine to leave many veterans perceiving that they have failed in the transition to civilian life when failure was never an option in the military. Veterans and families of veterans are at increased risk for issues of employment discrimination, job loss, and housing insecurity following transition out of the military and complications from these can lead to situations of homelessness for many veterans. Some of the most frequently cited reasons for housing insecurity among veterans and military families include: lack of affordable housing; limited income related to unemployment, often associated with transitioning out of the military with limited transferrable skills in the civilian labor market; lack of family and social support networks; effects from PTSD; and substance abuse as a maladaptive coping strategy. Social workers working with homeless veterans and military families assume that it is best to utilize a trauma-informed approach due to the high rates of traumatic events in military service.

Trauma-informed care is an intervention and organizational approach that focuses on how trauma may affect an individual's life and response to behavioral health services from prevention stages and throughout treatment. There are four key elements that a trauma-informed care approach incorporates and these include the following aspects: realizing the prevalence of trauma; recognizing how trauma affects all individuals involved with the program, organization, or system, including its own workforce; responding by putting this knowledge into practice; and actively taking measure to resist re-traumatizing clients in their work with them. The VHA works to help veterans secure housing through several programs in their efforts to move veterans and their families out of chronic patterns of homelessness through programs such as Health Care for Homeless Veterans (HCHV) and Supportive Services for Veterans and their Families (SSVF). The focus of these programs is to resolve housing crises as immediately as possible for veterans and their families. In addition to this, the goal of housing is through case management and referrals to health care and mental health treatment providers. Veterans receive services through case managers assigned to work closely with them and with landlords to negotiate plans and help with temporary financial assistance or subsidized housing vouchers for reduced monthly rent for veterans in need. The HUD/VASH Program is a partnership between the U.S. Department of Housing and Urban Development (HUD) and the U.S. Department of Veterans' Affairs Supported Housing Program (VASH). This program is comprised of a multidisciplinary team of VHA staff providing screening, case management, and supportive services including the HUD-VASH "Housing Choice" vouchers. The VHA's HUD/VASH program is also known as "social work boot camp" by many peer support specialists and social workers as this is often the entry point for new social workers entering into VHA careers who quickly learn the work. There is typically a high turnover rate at HUD/VASH programs and early or mid-career social workers often only stay in these positions for one year when they can apply for other positions across the VA that are only open to federal employees and not open to the public.

Some providers report that there is high burnout and compassion fatigue in these positions at the VHA because the work is very demanding due to limited social support networks in the veterans' lives, with often multiple and chronic crises, and needing to negotiate many non-profit organizations also working with the population. Many of the veterans who receive HUD/VASH assistance suffer from serious mental illness, substance abuse, and have limited family relationships due to attachment disruptions. These veterans often have no social safety nets to catch them if they face a significant housing crisis, food insecurity, legal involvement or court proceedings, or become destabilized emotionally. Social workers in HUD/VASH programs recommend having self-care routines, maintaining healthy boundaries with clients, knowing the shelter system in their local area, developing good time management skills, and being able to quickly assess and prioritize which crises need immediate attention as there are often multiple on a social worker's caseload. Many of the veteran clients in this program are homeless, have multiple risk factors, can be living in shelters, or are at risk for losing their housing situation. The Housing First Model is the focus of the work with decreasing the risk factors as the secondary longer-term work. The Harm Reduction Model is encouraged so that sobriety is not a requirement for housing vouchers for assistance in paying one's rent or associated housing bills. These programs are located in every city and state to provide emergency housing and shelter when veterans would otherwise be living in unsafe situations and/or need respite in situations of chronic, long-term homelessness.

Veteran Employment and Well-Being

The unemployment rate for veterans became a national concern in 2011 when Congress passed legislation to provide employment support and training to unemployed veterans and tax credits to private employers who hired veterans. In addition to the financial loss of income, long-term unemployment is often associated with housing insecurity and increased stress levels that also influence family functioning. Long-term unemployment is also associated with depression, irritability, decreased concentration and focus, demoralization, social isolation, and other problems that result from the lack of routine and structure (Tran et al., 2017). Studies comparing veterans to non-veteran peers found that veterans, especially younger veterans, are more likely to be unemployed than their civilian peers due to job loss incurred during separation from military service, and that this gap narrows with age and time since separation from active-duty military service (Loughran, 2014). The most recent data reported indicated that the average unemployment rate for both male and female veterans was just under 3% compared with non-veterans at 3.4% (Bureau of Labor Statistics [BLS], 2023). Unemployment rates for veterans by race and ethnicity in the same year were as follows: Black veterans 3.3% and Black non-veterans 5.6%; Asian veterans 2.7% and Asian non-veterans 2.8%; Hispanic/Latino veterans 2.9% and Hispanic/Latino non-veterans 4.9%; White veterans 2.7% and White non-veterans 3.2% (BLS, 2023). Labor statistics reported for 2022 included the following: the unemployment rate for all veterans was lower than the rate for non-veterans with unemployment rates for Black and White veterans lower than their non-veteran counterparts, and rates for Asian and Hispanic veterans not statistically different than their non-veteran counterparts. Among the 250,000 unemployed veterans, 54% were aged 25 to 54; 39% were aged 55 and over, and 7% were aged 18 to 24 years. Among post-9/11 veterans, those who reported a service-connected disability rating of less than 30% were much more likely to be in the labor force (95%) than those with a disability rating of 60% or higher (66%). The overall unemployment rate of veterans varied widely across states in the United States, ranging from 0.7% in North Dakota to 5.2% in Nevada (BLS, 2023).

Employment is a significant risk factor for consideration for veterans since unemployment can often lead to depression, and veterans have a greater risk for suicidal ideation when depressed than civilians do (Tran et al., 2016). One study reported that job loss is associated with negative changes in mental health functioning and that re-employment following unemployment results in improved mental health and well-being (Paul & Moser, 2009). When an adult family member is unemployed, household finances suffer, often leading to depleted savings, increased debt, difficulty with rent or mortgage payments, increased housing insecurity, increased family instability, and decreased family resiliency. Unemployment can lead to a host of negative psychological outcomes and one study found that unemployed female veterans were more likely to be depressed than female veterans who were employed (Hamilton et al., 2015).

Providers who assist newly separated veterans in their transition from active-duty military service to the civilian labor force can be helpful by preparing their clients for the possibility of being unemployed. Military families given the opportunity to discuss the factors that might accompany a period of sustained unemployment (such as the lack of structure, social isolation, or feelings of hopelessness) would be better equipped to manage such situations in adaptive ways if prepared for this possibility. In this way, education on the effects of unemployment might prevent some of the negative consequences and mental health problems associated with the often-difficult transition from military service to civilian employment, higher education, and community life following military service.

New Family Narratives Following Military Service

The transition and indoctrination into military culture is one that is rigid for service members but not for family members who have multiple, often confusing, choices for adopting the military-centered worldview and perspectives on life. The process for how one integrates their military-focused identity into their veteran/civilian identity is typically a major event in a service member and family's life course. The Double ABCX Adaptation to Stress model factors in the perception of this event (as a stressful situation) as a significant variable in the process that influences the outcome. As military children are often older teens or young adults by the time a military service member retires and the family transitions out of military service, the process often occurs at the same time that the military couple renegotiates their partner relationship. Questions such as where to live, where to work, and how close to be to extended family and/or adult children are typical decisions addressed during the transition out of military service.

Most of the literature on the transition process has focused on the veteran's experience as this has a concrete and definitive ending and is more visible to the outside observer of this process. In a process similar to the indoctrination into the military culture that occurs clearly for the veteran, and remains invisible for family members, the question of what to do with this part of one's cultural identity remains invisible and not well understood for the military family following military service. Since family members go through a transition process after military service, we can draw on the literature on the veteran's experience to guide our understanding of the experience of the military family. One of the most significant issues that comes up repeatedly in the literature on the veteran's experience following military service is the issue of adapting to the civilian way of life and integrating civilian values with established military values. The transition out of the military is often difficult the longer one has been in military service because the transition into the military typically occurs during young adulthood during the solidification of identity and personality. Young adults who enter military service and decide that it is not the right fit for them will often leave after one or two contracts and begin civilian lives. These individuals will still be in the stage of early adulthood and still in the process of forming their identity. The individuals who choose military service as a career or as a part-time career (NG/Reserves) will often proceed through middle adulthood with their military identity intact and may be at greater risk for more difficulties in the transition out due to the loss of this aspect of their identity. Military service members who have a long-term established identity that is based on military ethos and worldviews hold perceptions about daily living based on a strict set of expectations for behaviors, work ethics, and shared goals that are typically vastly different than those found in the civilian sector. In addition to the military way of life being uniquely different, in terms of being mission-driven with a sense of purpose, camaraderie, and trust fostered among its members, the level of one's identification with the military culture can influence outcomes in the process of establishing a new identity as part of the civilian world (Coll et al., 2012). In this way, Coll et al. (2012) point out that those who "over-identify" with the military culture are likely to experience challenges adapting to the civilian culture especially if they hold perceptions that the civilian world is inferior to the military one. Veterans who "under-identify" with the military culture often choose to actively do so as a means of easing their entry into new civilian roles and are likely to have less difficulty during the transition out of military service as a result (Coll et al., 2012).

When viewed through the lens of an adaptation to stress, the end of military service is a significant stressor in family life that all family members will go through in creating new individual and family narratives. The adaptation to a post-military civilian identity will be successful or not based on a number of factors including external resources, the service member and military family's level of identification with the military, and the perceptions held about civilians, the civilian ethos, and the civilian way of living. The aspect of the warrior society that contributes to these perceptions include the military's collectivist worldview and mindset where individual needs are subjugated for the "greater good" of the larger group's needs and sense of purpose in life. The military worldview is dialectically opposed to the civilian worldview in the United States where individual goals are highly regarded and often self-serving. In this way, the perceptions held about the civilian culture influence the transition process and relationships with civilian employers, colleagues, mental health providers, and neighbors in civilian living communities. While the military does an excellent job at the beginning of military service in the indoctrination process of new recruits into the military culture, worldview, and lifestyle, there is still much room for advancement in the transition process at the end of military service.

Veterans and Civilian Employment Challenges (Case Example)

John is a military veteran who served in active duty for 20 years and recently transitioned to the civilian workplace while navigating familiar but competing and stressful demands of a blended family, attending college at night, and working a full-time job in the civilian sector. His military training and experience had ingrained in him the value of being transparent as a member of a team for that team to function effectively and cohesively. As a result, he shared his experiences with his fellow students, college professors, colleagues, and supervisors at work. He did not hide or make any attempts at hiding his situation as he had been trained to do for the sake of the group as knowing what someone is going through is more helpful and safer for everyone than not knowing. He was often tired from lack of sleep with a recently adopted 18-month-old toddler waking up all hours while he was staying up late writing papers and as a result appeared exhausted both at work and in class, was easily distracted, and often irritable as a result. His civilian peers and supervisors did not understand this transparency and instead of communicating this directly, came to the inaccurate conclusion that he was suffering from PTSD from his military service. In addition to lacking knowledge about the military cultural value of transparency, his civilian peers attached the label that he was "a veteran with PTSD" and shared amongst themselves that they were scared of him. Instead of talking to him, they told their supervisor that they were scared to work with him and that the workplace had become a "hostile environment" for them as a result. His supervisor believed that he had no choice but to put John on administrative leave and proceeded to terminate his employment.

In addition to the suffering and loss of income for John and his family, this occurred based on a gross misperception by his civilian peers and his supervisor that he had PTSD. The practice of terminating someone's employment based on a perception of a disability that is not true is illegal and if substantiated, John would be compensated, his employment reinstated, and any/all government contracts with the organization would be withdrawn and business never conducted with that company again. All these painful events could have been easily prevented through a civilian cultural competency training offered by the employer. Similar protections are in place in institutions of higher education although they tend to be more complicated in terms of student veterans and the paths that are taken and navigated.

> The Uniformed Services Employment and Reemployment Rights Act (USERRA) and Title I of the Americans with Disabilities Act (ADA) protect veterans from employment discrimination. Title I of the ADA prohibits an employer from treating an applicant or employee unfavorably in all aspects of employment—including hiring, promotions, job assignments, training, termination, and any other terms, conditions, and privileges of employment—because he or she has a disability, a history of having a disability, or because the employer regards him as having a disability. That means, for example, that it is illegal for an employer to refuse to hire a veteran because the veteran has PTSD, was previously diagnosed with PTSD, or because the employer assumes the veteran has PTSD.
>
> (United States Equal Employment Opportunity Commission, 2020)

Appendix

Self-Assessment for Military Family Resiliency (for Family Members)

- List your core family values (identify and name 3–5 of these):

  ____

  ____

- Family motto/mission statement to describe your family (briefly in a few words):

  ____

  ____

- Parenting styles: describe your parenting style (together if partnered and in individual ways) and how you have managed lengthy separations such as during deployments in terms of the attachment and bond between family members. Describe whether the nature of your parenting style changes during times of distress or separations that are stressful for your family and if so, in what ways does it change?

  ____

  ____

  ____

- Family perceptions (choose any of the following ways that thinking about problems) may be limiting or strengthening your family's resiliency:
- Rigid or flexible thinking
- Concrete or shades of grey thinking
- Catastrophic or multiple levels of distress of problems
- Forgetting or honoring strengths
- Forgetting or appropriately using humor
- Others not listed:

  ____

- Family coping and adaptation (name one way in which your family coped/adapted well to a problem or a stressful situation in the past):

  ____

  ____

- Strengths as a team (identify/name 3–5 of your family strengths at working together to solve problems):

  ____

  ____

  ____

- Traumatic triggers (identify topics or behaviors in your family that are triggers for other family members and lead to emotional outbursts such as crying/anger or behaviors such as storming out of the room/house or withdrawing/shutting down):

  ____

  ____

  ____

- Interpersonal boundaries (identify situations in your family where individual boundaries may get blurry and individual wants/needs are difficult to express/maintain):

  ____

  ____

  ____

Cultural Humility Self-Assessment (for Civilian Providers working with Military/Veteran Clients)

A cultural humility self-assessment tool is often located as grounding between cross-cultural practice frameworks to improve self-awareness and clinical treatment practices among mental health providers. This questionnaire helps guide clinicians working with veterans and military-connected populations in improved clinical interventions and effective treatments.

1 Many veteran clients at the VHA report having a new treatment provider every year and often have to repeat their stories to civilian providers who are in training roles or clinical internships.

   1.1. *Have you ever worked with veterans and were unfamiliar with the culture? How did you address this in the treatment initially and over time?*
   1.2. *If you have been in this role, how did you feel? How did it make the client feel being in the role of teacher about this aspect of their life?*
   1.3. *If you have had conversations about this, who initiated these and what impact did they have on your working relationship and the treatment in general?*

2 Many clients have reported that mental health providers do not maintain eye contact during sessions despite the importance of this in building rapport and establishing trust.

   2.1. *Have you ever found yourself avoiding eye contact with your clients and if so, why did this happen? What was going on in the session that led you and/or your client to avoid eye contact?*
   2.2. *How could you discuss this issue in terms of tolerating discomfort and strengthening working alliance/attachment when it might be uncomfortable to do so?*

3 Some military/veteran clients have reported that they hesitate to disclose feelings surrounding moral injury with civilian mental health providers.

   3.1. *Have you ever felt that your military/veteran clients were reluctant to share important information with you and if so, were you able to address this directly?*

3.2. *Have you ever felt unsure of how to proceed during a session when the topic of moral injury, or morally injurious events, came up? If so, did you address this directly at the time, talk to a colleague/supervisor afterwards, or let the topic go without returning to it in the next session to allow the client to decide?*
3.3. *Do you know the definition of moral injury and the difference between moral injury and posttraumatic stress well enough to be able to introduce/explore it in treatment sessions?*
3.4. *Do you feel comfortable discussing issues of morality and moral injury from war? Do you think there is an optimal point in time in treatment to discuss these issues (such as at intake, in couples/group treatments, or wait for the client to raise it)? What contextual factors would make these discussions easier in general?*

4 Some military/veteran clients have reported wanting therapy that includes unstructured treatment sessions that do not follow a script or an evidence-based manual.

4.1. *How often do you initiate therapeutic conversations with your military/veteran clients that are not evidence-based practices?*
4.2. *In your experience, is it more or less effective when you have unstructured therapy sessions with your military/veteran clients?*

Pre-Deployment Case Study: The Military Family Stable at Home

Case Study: The Drako Family During the Pre-Deployment Phase

Danielle is a 15-year-old girl living at Ft. Levenworth, Kansas with her mother, father, and her younger brothers who are 8 and 4 years old. Her father, John, is a Marine who had returned from a deployment to an undisclosed location in the Middle East last year. They have just received PCS orders to Virginia in six months as her father has been transferred and will be deployed again. This is his third deployment in the past six years. John grew up in a military family and lived through his father's military life, also a Marine, and being deployed twice during his childhood. Danielle was 8–9 years old during her father's first deployment to Iraq, 14 years old during his second deployment to Afghanistan, and will be 16 years old for this last tour. Danielle just finished her freshman year of high school and has a boyfriend for the first time in her life. She is experiencing "mood swings" according to her mother, Jane. She has outbursts of irritability and anger combined with periods of being in love with her boyfriend and euphoric about her relationships in general. At times, Danielle gets very clingy with her mother and seems to regress to earlier childhood stages, even curling up next to mom on the couch and sucking her thumb, wanting to cuddle together while watching TV. Her mother often resents this behavior and tells her she needs to "just grow up" and walks away. Her mother describes Danielle as always having been a "needy child" who had trouble separating from her and never having many friends outside of the family. Danielle always had difficulty with the moves and changes to new schools because she was shy and socially uncomfortable by nature.

This past year, Danielle became defiant and rebellious, staying out past her curfew, smoking marijuana, and drinking beer with her friends and her boyfriend in a parking lot by the mall off base. Her mother says that she has continued to test limits with her as a parent. Her mother reported feeling guilty that Danielle was going through such a tough time and that she began to buy her gifts during the last deployment to make her feel better. Danielle starting hanging out with this new group of friends shortly after her father's R&R vacation at home for two weeks last summer. It was the first time she had a group of friends in her life and drinking beer and smoking marijuana helped her to relax and be social when she didn't feel that way. All of the teens in this group were arrested recently for disorderly conduct and possession of marijuana. They were released because there was no basis to keep them as none of them were dealing drugs and most of them were young. Her father's reaction was to enforce stricter curfews, rules, and consequences. He became disappointed and angry at her; as a result, there is now a great deal of conflict between them about this group and her behavior. Danielle had been angry at her father following his return home from deployment, and they were having increased difficulty communicating before the recent arrest. Danielle's mother expressed feelings of having done something wrong in her parenting, since she was single parenting for three years when she counted up the months alone and blames herself for the problems that Danielle has experienced in her development. She has been pulling away from Danielle since her husband returned and told him she was handing the tasks of raising Danielle over to him to do a "better job," focusing instead on her sons whom she thinks she can be a better mother to since they are still so young. The youngest boy, Dylan, has refused to be alone with John since he returned from his last deployment and won't go anywhere without Jane. The older son, Charlie, has been having trouble at school and his grades have been slipping this past year to C's and D's, in addition to getting into fights on the playground with other boys over rules in their games and who's playing fair and who's cheating to win. These fights escalated to the point of Charlie's suspension from school on multiple occasions.

Jane had an affair during the second deployment. The family had moved from Hawaii to San Diego where John was stationed at Camp Pendleton. Danielle was 12 years old and in a new middle school. Her parents had many arguments when her father returned home and found out about the affair. One argument escalated into a physical fight that Danielle got in the middle of while trying to break up and stop the fight. Following that incident, Danielle began having trouble sleeping, developed difficulty concentrating in school, and her grades began to suffer. She became the focus of her parents' arguments at home. Jane's reason for having the affair was that she was lonely and depressed at the time and with a history of depression during the post-partum period following Danielle's birth, Jane feared the depression would return if she didn't do something like having the affair. Jane worried that she would be unable to take care of all that she needed to in terms of parenting and home responsibilities. She says she did this to keep the family together, for the emotional connection to someone other than the children, and not for the physical part which was there as well. John is confused about her reasoning but feels so guilty for having left her so many times that he doesn't feel he can argue about it much.

Before Jane was born, her father had been a Captain in the Army in Vietnam. Jane never talked about her father's service in the Army throughout her childhood, and she is still reluctant to do so, other than to agree with her mother that it had occurred whenever she brings it up. Jane remembers the feeling of "walking on eggshells" around her father all the time. She feels this impacted her greatly in terms of making her an anxious child. She also had difficulty making friends because she says she was embarrassed to have friends over to the house because her father's moods were so unpredictable, and he had emotional outbursts at random times. As a result, Jane does not want her children to grow up this way and feels it's important to stand up to John in ways her mother did not stand up to her father. Danielle's strengths include being very artistic and creative; she plays guitar, writes, and sings her own songs when she is upset to calm herself down. She is very empathic with her mother and understands her mother's feelings and reactions.

She feels a close connection with her mother that she doesn't feel with her father. She has often assumed the role of caretaker to her younger brothers when her mother was overwhelmed or needed her help with parenting during the deployments and has become a certified babysitter for neighborhood children, making some extra money in her spare time.

Case Study Discussion: The Drako Family during the Pre-Deployment Phase

The family system operates from a biopsychosocial perspective that details all the family members across three generations which adds to a deeper understanding of the historical context of the system as well as the intergenerational transmission of stress and risk factors. The history of the military service member's involvement with the military begins their story, together with their reasons for joining being due to a family of service members and the generational tradition of military service. The military couple has both risk and resiliency factors as well as the adolescent daughter who struggles with depression and substance use as a means of coping with stress. All the children have systemic risk factors present in the family system that tends to become overwhelmed in the presence of strong emotions that are difficult to manage. There are several academic and social risk factors from the multiple school changes and geographic relocations, undiagnosed learning disabilities, and mental health conditions that are contributing factors leading to behavioral adaptations to these risk factors causing stress for the entire family system.

Deployment Case Study: The Military Family Adapts to Loss and Upheaval

Case Study: The Drako Family During the Deployment Phase

Shortly after John left for his deployment, Jane found out that Danielle had been sleeping with her boyfriend and they began having repeated arguments about it. Jane had pulled away from her daughter when John was home and now that he was gone again, Danielle had no one to turn to in terms of being attached to either of her parents. Danielle turned to her boyfriend for the attention and comfort she was seeking instead and became overly attached to him, rejecting her old friends and relying on him for all her social support. This boyfriend, Mark, eventually pulled away from her as well and broke up with her for that reason, calling her immature and needy, telling her that he couldn't make her happy. Danielle became depressed and began to self-harm, cutting her arms superficially at first but growing in intensity over the first six months of the deployment. Jane found out about it from the guidance counselor at school who Danielle had gone to speak with because her grades were falling, she felt out of control in general, and was scared most of the time that she would really hurt herself one day. Danielle presented as needy yet shy and aloof at the same time to most people, making it almost impossible for her to get her needs for emotional connection and attachment met, without the use of substances which was becoming more and more often. The guidance counselor has made a positive connection with Danielle and this has been helping her get through going to school every day and stay motivated to keep trying to get good grades. The counselor enrolled her in a "friendship group" at school where six students each lunch together once/week and talk about things bothering them. There is one girl who was chosen for the group as a "strength" in the group as a role model and has invited Danielle to go to the movies with her twice so far which was a lot of fun for Danielle.

Jane began therapy during the deployment because she had also become depressed and overwhelmed by the stress of parenting three children as a single mother. She had no emotional resources to take care of Danielle's needs that were growing increasingly greater every day. Her therapist was recommending family therapy for her and Danielle together but Jane didn't want to until John came home because she was angry that she was carrying the burden. Jane didn't understand why Danielle acted so aloof and uninterested in the family and decided that she wasn't really that motivated to be a part of family life. The older boy, Charlie, became a parentified child in the family and assumed the roles that John had held in the family such as taking care of the dogs, taking out the garbage, and checking in on Jane's emotional life every day. Charlie had many friends but chose to stay home with Jane most of his free time rather than go out with them on the weekends or after school. He would stay up late watching TV with Jane so she didn't get too lonely and helped take care of his younger brother, Dylan, in terms of babysitting and making lunches for him in the mornings so she could sleep in late as they got ready for school. He was very competent at all of these chores and felt proud of being able to fill his father's shoes in terms of taking care of his mother and brother, which his father had told him to do in his absence.

Case Study Discussion: Adjusting to Loss and Managing Deployment Separation

The family managed the upheaval of deployment separation and the loss of the military service member from the family system. All of the various roles and responsibilities previously held by the service member have been redistributed to other family members as the family system needs to restructure itself to manage all of the tasks of daily living. The family system and individual members decide and communicate in spoken and unspoken ways who takes on which roles, how this is decided, and challenges faced when members do not believe other family members are living up to expectations. Communication with the service member during the long-term separation keeps that person involved in daily life for many families. This family's choice to exclude the service member from daily life and major decision-making has benefits and tolls to the system as a whole. In this situation, communication between home and deployment becomes static and remains on a superficial level which all members agree to either outwardly or by default of not wanting to "rock the boat" in terms of patterns that are established by the couple/parents in the system. This superficial pattern of communicating between the family at-home and the service member leads to anxiety for family members navigating separate lives during the deployment as the deployment stress is weighing on all family members on a daily basis and the question remains of whether or not to convey these situations during brief weekly phone calls. Nothing of significance is being communicated in either direction (from home or deployment) in this phase of the case study although there are multiple situations of crisis and significance occurring in both places that are not shared or expressed emotionally. The outcome of the extended period of superficial and false communication over the course of one year leads the family to fall into the habit of this type of communication process. The risk for this family is whether or not they will be able to change this style of communicating when the deployment ends and the service member returns home to the family and everyone needs to communicate in completely different ways again.

Post-Deployment Case Study: The Military Family Accommodates to Change

Case Study: The Drako Family During the Reintegration Phase

John returned home following a nine-month deployment where he sustained several blast injuries from IEDs that his vehicle had hit while on the road, the last one with loss of consciousness. He was medically evacuated to LRMC for IED explosion with LOC of 20 minutes. He presents with irritability, being socially isolated, ruminating thoughts of self-blame due to missions downrange, nightmares, tremors triggered by anxiety, dissociative episodes, flashbacks, foreshortened sense of the future, and difficulty focusing and concentrating. He demonstrates impulsivity and impaired judgement, which restrict his ability to drive, and assume other related responsibilities. Jake's medical conditions include tinnitus, five plaques in his brain, and degenerative disc disease at L-4 causing lower back pain and hip issues.

Treatment has included individual cognitive processing therapy, a group-based intensive outpatient program for PTSD, OT services for TBI, and Botox injections for migraines on a monthly basis. Jake's medications include Prozac, Prazosin, Adderall, benzodiazepines, and sleep medications. He received a permanent profile for PTSD, post-concussive syndrome, and degenerative disc disease. He is in the process of being medically retired from the military and needs to find a new job and career as soon as he can. Daniella is having difficulty tolerating the "new normal" as John is not able to fulfill the same roles and routines that he had done previously. John is not able to drive the children to school or after-school activities, he cannot be in public spaces that might be loud or brightly lit due to his migraines and posttraumatic stress, and stopped being intimate shortly after his return home. John has difficulty sleeping longer than two hours at a time, has frequent nightmares that cause him to lash out in his sleep and he once hit Danielle while she was sleeping, which has led to his sleeping on the couch at night. Danielle feels overwhelmed by the current situation and is becoming depressed and withdrawn from John and the family. She has returned to her therapist for weekly individual sessions and has been questioning whether the incident of being hit in her sleep is domestic violence or not because it has triggered her posttraumatic stress from the previous incident of domestic violence that the couple had sustained.

Danielle has withdrawn from the family and is making plans to join the military once she graduates from high school. She feels badly for her parents but decided that she could not help them and moved on to helping herself instead; she barely speaks to either of her parents and is only home to eat, sleep, and shower on most days. Charlie is 10 years old and continues to struggle academically and socially with his peers in school, having developed impulse control problems and difficulty reading social cues. Dylan, who is 5 years old, has been having increased generalized anxiety, difficulty sleeping at night, and nightly bedwetting incidents. Dylan has been sleeping with Danielle since John began sleeping on the couch, and developed school phobia, demanding to stay home most days, and his teacher wants him to repeat kindergarten next year as a result.

Case Study Discussion: Managing Reintegration Stress

The Drako family in the post-deployment period begins to manage the grey area of family life with the introduction of unresolved posttraumatic stress as they adjust and accommodate to the avoidance, intrusion, and arousal symptoms that John exhibits in daily life. These accommodations are how the family seeks and preserves a sense of stability for the system to survive by colluding with denial of the stress. The family system is forced to accommodate to the presence of ongoing behaviors of social avoidance, anger, depression, and alcohol use as individual family members manage stress reactions.

The case study will examine how the adaptations that are made to the return of the service member, and to the new stress in the previously stable family system, are understood in terms of repetitive, yet unsuccessful, attempts by all family members to return the system to previous levels of stability. As the family remains destabilized and does not return to a stable functioning system, the service member/veteran and spouse experiences a sense of confusion about what is going on in their relationship and a loss for words to explain it to their children or themselves. The daily presence of traumatic stress and the family's reaction of approaching and avoiding difficult and overwhelming emotions leads to individual family members detaching from one another. This process results in ambiguous loss that leads to role ambiguity in the system as the veteran and all family members struggle to return to previous roles in the family but cannot do so. The family experiences that it is not possible for them to return to previous family functioning and miss the emotional connections they once had with each other. The military couple experience loss in the attachment they once held and conflict emerges in the relationship. Both individuals experience a sense of isolation in the marriage but cope with these feelings because approaching them usually ends in conflict and chaos for the entire family. As a result, they have lost their previous roles, and the ensuing role ambiguity opens up channels for all family members to experience secondary traumatic stress. The family learns through counselling to think in flexible ways to create a new family narrative and adjust their family system to remain hopeful for the future.

The family reaches a breaking point, however, when the adaptations to the changes do not work over time and the couple considers divorce as a solution to what has become an untenable situation in the family's home life. The family comes to understand this through dialog with a mental health provider who explains what has been happening in the family system and offers tools for tolerating distressing feelings, setting healthy boundaries, and solving family problems together in a collaborative manner. The provider describes how adaptations worked to keep the system stable initially but were maladaptive over time as the family needed to grieve the loss of the previous system (family) and define how the new system (family) could be strong. Although it would be different, it was still a family to be proud through the very resilient nature of all of the family members.

Bibliography

Acion, L., Ramirez, M. R., Jorge, R. E., & Arndt, S. (2013). Substance use among military children. *Addiction*, 108, 1418–1425. https://doi.org/10.1111/add.12161.

Adler-Baeder, F., Pittman, J. F., Taylor, L., & Pasley, K. (2005). *Marital transitions in military families: Their prevalence and relevance for adaptation to the military (final report)*. West Lafayette, Indiana: Military Family Research Institute, Purdue University.

Ainsworth, M. S. (1989). Attachments beyond infancy. *American Psychologist*, 44(4), 709.

Aleman-Tovar, J., Schraml-Block, K., DiPietro-Wells, R. et al. (2022). Exploring the advocacy experiences of military families with children who have disabilities. *Journal of Child & Family Studies*, 31, 843–853. https://doi.org/10.1007/s10826-021-02161-5.

American Psychiatric Association (2013). *Diagnostic and statistical manual of mental disorders: DSM-5* (Vol. 5, No. 5). Washington, DC: American Psychiatric Association.

Anyiwo, N., Palmer, G. J., Garrett, J. M., Starck, J. G., & Hope, E. C. (2020). Racial and political resistance: An examination of the sociopolitical action of racially marginalized youth. *Current Opinion in Psychology*, 35, 86–91.

Aronson K. R., Kyler S. J., Moeller J. D., & Perkins D.F. (2016). Understanding military families who have dependents with special health care and/or educational needs. *Disability and Health Journal*, 9(3), 423–430.

Bannink, F. P. (2007). Solution-focused brief therapy. *Journal of Contemporary Psychotherapy*, 37, 87–94.

Basham, K. (2008). Homecoming as safe haven or the new front: Attachment and detachment in military couples. *Clinical Social Work Journal*, 36, 83–96.

Berger, N., Bonuck, E. R., Taber, K. H., Kalvin, C., Dolber, T., & Cristian, A. (2011). Multifamily group treatment for veterans with traumatic brain injury. *Professional Psychology: Research and Practice*, 42(1), 70–78. https://doi.org/10.1037/a0022319.

Bjornestad, A., Schweinle, A., & Elhai, J. (2014). Measuring secondary traumatic stress symptoms in military spouses with the posttraumatic stress disorder checklist military version. *The Journal of Nervous and Mental Disease*, 202(12), 864–869.

Blamey, H., & Phillips, A. (2019). The impact of parental military service on child well-being. *Journal of Military, Veteran, and Family Health*. https://jmvfh.utpjournals.press/doi/10.3138/jmvfh.2019-0014.

Bobrow, J., Cook, E., Knowles, C., & Vieten, C. (2013). Coming all the way home: Integrative community care for those who serve. *Psychological Services*, 10(2), 137–144. https://doi.org/10.1037/a0031279.

Booth, B., Falk, W. W., Segal, D. R., & Segal, M. W. (2000). The impact of military presence in local labor markets on the employment of women. *Gender and Society*, 14(2), 318–322.

Borah, E., & Fina, B. (2017). Military spouses speak up: A qualitative study of military and veteran spouses' perspectives. *Journal of Family Social Work*, 20(2), 144–161.

Boss, P. (2009). *Ambiguous loss: Learning to live with unresolved grief*. Harvard University Press.

Boss, P. (2007). Ambiguous loss theory: Challenges for scholars and practitioners. *Family Relations*, 56(2), 105–111.

Boss, P. (2006). *Loss, trauma, and resilience: Therapeutic work with ambiguous loss*. New York: W.W. Norton.

Boss, P. (2002). *Family stress management: A contextual approach*. Thousand Oaks: CA, Sage.

Boss, P. (1999). *Ambiguous loss: Learning to live with unresolved grief*. Cambridge, MA: Harvard Press.

Bowen, G. L., Mancini, J. A., Martin, J. A., Ware, W. B., & Nelson, J. P. (2003). Promoting the adaptation of military families: An empirical test of a community practice model. *Family Relations*, 52(1), 33–44. https://doi.org/10.1111/j.1741-3729.2003.00033.

Bowers, E. P., John Geldhof, G., Johnson, S. K., Lerner, J. V., & Lerner, R. M. (2014). Special issue introduction: Thriving across the adolescent years: A view of the issues. *Journal of Youth and Adolescence*, 43, 859–868.

Bowlby, J. (1980). *Attachment and loss. Volume* III. *Loss: Sadness and depression*. Hogarth.

Bowlby, J. (1973). *Attachment and loss. Volume* II*: Separation: anxiety and anger*. New York, NY: Basic Books.

Bowlby, J. (1969). *Attachment and loss. Volume* I. Random House.

Bowlby, J., & Ainsworth, M. (2013). The origins of attachment theory. *Attachment Theory: Social, Developmental, and Clinical Perspectives*, 45(28), 759–775.

Bradbard, D. A., Maury, R., & Armstrong, N. J. (2016, November). *The force behind the force: Case profiles of successful military spouses balancing employment, service, and family* (Employing Military Spouses, Paper No. 2). Syracuse, NY: Institute for Veterans and Military Families, Syracuse University.

Brown, R. P., & Lee, M. N. (2005). *Stigma consciousness and the race gap in college academic achievement. Self and Identity*, 4, 149–157.

Bryan, C. J., Bryan, A. O., Roberge, E., Leifker, F. R., & Rozek, D. C. (2018). Moral injury, posttraumatic stress disorder, and suicidal behavior among National Guard personnel. *Psychological Trauma: Theory, Research, Practice, and Policy*, 10(1), 36–45.

Bryant-Davis, T., & Wong, E. (2013). Faith to move mountains: Religious coping, spirituality, and interpersonal trauma recovery. *American Psychologist*, 68(8), 675–684.

Buehrle, J. (2014). "Us" as the United States: sparking community-based solutions for supporting military-connected children and their families. *Children & Schools*, 36(1), https://doi.org/10.1093/cs/cdt045.

Bureau of Labor Statistics (2023). U.S. Department of Labor. Retrieved from: www.bls.gov/news.release/pdf/vet.pdf.

Burke, J., & Miller, A. R. (2016). The effects of military change of station moves on spousal earnings. Working Paper: RAND National Defense Research Institute. www.rand.org/content/dam/rand/pubs/working_papers/WR1100/WR1170/RAND_WR1170.pdf

Canfield, J. (2019). Civilian spousal employment. In E. L. Weiss & C. A. Castro (Eds.), *American military life in the 21st century: Social, cultural, and economic issues and trends*. Santa Barbara, CA: ABC-CLIO, LLC. (Vol. 2, pp. 360–372).

Canfield, J. (2014). Traumatic stress and affect management in military families. *Social Work in Mental Health*, 12(5–6), 544–559.

Canfield, J., & Weiss, E. (2015). Integrating military and veteran culture in social work education: Implications for curriculum inclusion. *Journal of Social Work Education, 51*(sup1), S128–S144.

Carr, M. M., Potenza, M. N., Serowik, K. L., & Pietrzak, R. H. (2021). Race, ethnicity, and clinical features of alcohol use disorder among US military veterans: Results from the national health and resilience in veterans study. *American Journal of Addiction*, 30, 26–33.

Carroll, J. S., Olson, C. D., & Buckmiller, N. (2007). Family boundary ambiguity: A 30-year review of theory, research, and measurement. *Family Relations*, 56, 210–230.

Castaneda, L. W. and M. C. Harrell (2008). Military spouse employment: A grounded theory approach to experiences and perceptions. *Armed Forces & Society*, 34(3), 389–412.

Castro, C. A., Kintzle, S., & Hassan, A. M. (2015). The combat veteran paradox: Paradoxes and dilemmas encountered with reintegrating combat veterans and the agencies that support them. *Traumatology*, 21(4), 299.

Catalano, R. F., Berglund, M. L., Ryan, J. A., Lonczak, H. S., & Hawkins, J. D. (2004). Positive youth development in the United States: Research findings on evaluations of positive youth development programs. *The Annals of the American Academy of Political and Social Science*, 591(1), 98–124.

Chandra, A., Lara-Cinisomo, S., Jaycox, L. H., Tanielian, T., Burns, R. M., Ruder, T., & Han, B. (2010). Children on the homefront: The experience of children from military families. *Pediatrics*, 125(1), 16–25.

Charach, A., Yeung, E., Climans, T., & Lillie, E. (2011). Childhood attention-deficit/hyperactivity disorder and future substance use disorders: comparative meta-analyses. *Journal of the American Academy of Child & Adolescent Psychiatry*, 50(1), 9–21.

Coll, J. E., Weiss, E. L., & Metal, M. (2013). Military culture and diversity. In: A. Rubin, E. L. Weiss, & J. E. Coll (Eds). *Handbook of military social work* (pp. 21–36). Hoboken, NJ: Wiley & Sons.

Coll, J. E., Weiss, E. L., Draves, P., & Dyer, D. (2012). The impact of military cultural awareness, experience, attitudes, and education on clinician self-efficacy in the treatment of veterans. *Journal of International Continuing Social Work Education*, 15(1), 39–48.

Cooke, Thomas J., & Karen Speirs. (2005). Migration and Employment among the Civilian Spouses of Military Personnel. *Social Science Quarterly*, 86(2), 343–355.

Cooney, R., De Angelis, K., & Segal, M. W. (2011). Moving with the military: Race, class, and gender differences in the employment consequences of tied migration. *Race, Gender & Class*, 18 (1–2),360–384.

Cozza, C. S. J., & Lerner, R. M. (2013). Military children and families: Introducing the issue. *The Future of Children*, 23(2), 3–11.

Cunradi C. B. (2009). Intimate partner violence among Hispanic men and women: The role of drinking, neighborhood disorder, and acculturation-related factors. *Violence and Victims*, 24(1), 83–97. https://doi.org/10.1891/0886-6708.24.1.83.

Davis, E. E. (2014, April). Current knowledge about military-connected children with special health care needs and their families. In *Military-connected children with special health care needs and their families* (pp. 6–13). Bethesda, MD: Symposium conducted at the National Institute of Child Health and Human Development (NICHD) and the HSC Foundation. www.nichd.nih.gov/sites/default/files/about/meetings/2014/Documents/military_families_summary.pdf.

De Angelis, K., & Segal, M. W. (2015). Transitions in the military and the family as greedy institutions: Original concept and current applicability. In R. Moelke, M. Andres, & P. Manigart (Eds.), *Military families and war in the 21st century* (pp. 22–42). Routledge.

Defense Manpower Data Center (2013). *2012 Survey of active duty spouses: Tabulations of responses*. Report No. 2013–2017. Washington, D.C., DMDC.

Defense Manpower Data Center (2007). *2006 Survey of active duty spouses: Administration, datasets, and codebook*. Arlington, VA: U.S. Department of Defense. Retrieved from www.esd.whs.mil /Portals/54/Documents /FOID/Reading%20Room /Personnel_Related /2006_ADSS_Codebook _and_Appendices_A-M-but_not_H.pdf.

Defense Suicide Prevention Office (2014). Department of defense suicide event report CY 2014. www.dspo. mil/Portals/113/Documents/CY%202014%20DoDSER%20 Annual%20Report% 20-%20Final.pdf.

Dekel, R., Solomon, Z., & Bleich, A. (2005) Emotional distress and marital adjustment of caregivers: Contribution of level of impairment and appraised burden. *Anxiety, Stress, & Coping*, 18 (1), 71–82, doi:10.1080/10615800412336427.

Department of Defense (2013). *2013 Military demographics: Profile of the military community*. Washington, DC: Office of the Deputy Assistant Secretary of Defense (Military Community and Family Policy).

de Shazer, S., & Berg, I. K. (1997). “What works?” Remarks on research aspects of solution-focused brief therapy. *Journal of Family Therapy*, 19(2), 121–124.

Donoho, C. J., LeardMann, C., O’Malley, C. A., Walter, K. H., Riviere, L. A., Curry, J. F., & Adler, A. B. (2018). Depression among military spouses: Demographic, military, and service member psychological health risk factors. *Depression and Anxiety*, 35(12), 1137–1144.

Ebaugh, H. R. F. (1988). *Becoming an ex: The process of role exit*. Chicago: University of Chicago Press.

Erikson, E. H. (1982). *The life cycle completed*. New York: Norton.

Evans, L., McHugh, T., Hopwood, M. and Watt, C. (2003). Chronic posttraumatic stress disorder and family functioning of Vietnam veterans and their partners. *Australian and New Zealand Journal of Psychiatry*, 37, 765–772. https://doi.org/10.1111/j.1440-1614.2003.01267.x.

Exum, H., Coll, J. E., & Weiss, E. L. (2011). *A civilian counselor's primer for counseling veterans* (2nd Ed.). Deerpark, NY: Linus Publications, Inc.

Franz, M. R., Sanders, W., Nillni, Y. I., Vogt, D., Matteo, R., & Galovski, T. (2022). PTSD and parental functioning: The protective role of neighborhood cohesion among Black and White veterans. *Psychological Trauma: Theory, Research, Practice, and Policy*, 14, S4–S12. https://doi.org/10.1037/tra0001123.

Galovski, T., & Lyons, J. A. (2004). Psychological sequelae of combat violence: A review of the impact of PTSD on the veteran's family and possible interventions. *Aggression and Violent Behavior*, 9(5), 477–501.

Gambardella, L. C. (2008). Role-exit theory and marital discord following extended military deployment. *Perspectives in Psychiatric Care*, 44, 169–174.

Gerlock, A. A., Grimesey, J., & Sayre, G. (2014). Military-related posttraumatic stress disorder and intimate relationship behaviors: A developing dyadic relationship model. *Journal of Marital and Family Therapy*, 40, 344–356.

Goin-Kochel, R. P., Meyers, B. J., & Mackintosh, V. G. (2007). Parental reports on the use of treatments and therapies for children with autism spectrum disorders. *Research in Autism Spectrum Disorders*, 1, 195–209. https://doi.org/10.1016/j.rasd.2006.08.006.

Gonzalez, G., Matthews, L. J., Posard, M., Roshan, P., & Ross, S. M. (2015). Evaluation of the military spouse employment partnership: Progress report on first stage of analysis (p. 70). RAND Corporation.

Gray, M. J., Schorr, Y., Nash, W., Lebowitz, L., Amidon, A., Lansing, A., ... Litz, B. T. (2012). Adaptive disclosure: An open trial of a novel exposure based intervention for service members with combat-related psychological stress injuries. *Behavior Therapy*, 43(2), 407–415.

Green, S., Nurius, P. S., & Lester, P. (2013). Spouse psychological well-being: A keystone to military family health. *Journal of Human Behavior in the Social Environment*, 23(6), 753–768.

Hall, L. K. (2016). *Counseling military families: What mental health professionals need to know*. Routledge.

Hamilton, A. B., Williams, L., & Washington, D. L. (2015). Military and mental health correlates of unemployment in a national sample of women veterans. *Medical Care*, 53, S32–S38.

Harrell, M. C., Lim, N., Castaneda, L. W., & Golinelli, D. (2004). *Working around the military: Challenges to military spouse employment and education*. Santa Monica, Calif.: RAND, MG-196-OSD.

Harrington-LaMorie, J., Jordan, J. R., Ruocco, K., & Cerel, J. (2018). Surviving families of military suicide loss: Exploring postvention peer support. *Death Studies*, 42(3), 143–154. https://doi.org/10.1080/07481187.2017.1370789.

Herzog, J. R., Whitworth, J. D., & Scott, D. L. (2020). Trauma informed care with military populations. *Journal of Human Behavior in the Social Environment*, 30(3), 265–278.

Hill, R. (1949). *Families under stress: Adjustment to the crises of war separation and reunion*. New York, NY: Harper & Brothers.

Hoge, C. W., Ivany, C. G., & Adler, A. B. (2017). Suicidal behaviors within army units: Contagion and implications for public health interventions. *JAMA Psychiatry*, 74(9), 871–872. https://doi.org/10.1001/jamapsychiatry.2017.1908.

Hook, J. N., Davis, D. E., Owen, J., Worthington, E. L., Jr., & Utsey, S. O. (2013). Cultural humility: Measuring openness to culturally diverse clients. *Journal of Counseling Psychology*, 60(3), 353–366.

Hope, E. C., Velez, G., Offidani-Bertrand, C., Keels, M., & Durkee, M. I. (2018). Political activism and mental health among Black and Latinx college students. *Cultural Diversity and Ethnic Minority Psychology*, 24(1), 26.

Hope, E. C., Keels, M., & Durkee, M. I. (2016). Participation in Black Lives Matter and deferred action for childhood arrivals: Modern activism among Black & Latino college students. *Journal of Diversity in Higher Education*, 9, 203–215.

Hosek, J., & Wadsworth, S. M. (2013). Economic conditions of military families. *The Future of Children*, 23(2), 41–59.

Hosek, J., Asch, B. J., Fair, C. C., Martin, C., & Mattock, M. (2002). *Married to the military: The employment and earnings of military wives compared with those of civilian wives*. Santa Monica, Calif.: Rand Corporation.

Huebner, A. J., & Mancini, J.A. (2005). *Adjustment among adolescents in military families when a parent is deployed: A final report submitted to the Military Family Research Institute and the Department of Defense Quality of Life Office*. Falls Church, Virginia: Virginia Tech, Department of Human Development.

Huebner, A. J., Mancini, J. A., Bowen, G. L., & Orthner, D. K. (2009). Shadowed by war: Building community capacity to support military families. *Family Relations*, 58(2), 216–228.

Hughes, D. A. (2007). *Attachment-focused family therapy*. New York: WW Norton & Company.

Hwang, W. C., & Goto, S. (2008). The impact of perceived racial discrimination on the mental health of Asian American and Latino college students. *Cultural Diversity and Ethnic Minority Psychology*, 14(4), 326.

Johnson, S. M. (2019). *Attachment theory in practice: Emotionally focused therapy (EFT) with individuals, couples, and families*. New York: Guilford Publications.

Kamarck, K. N. (2019). *Diversity, inclusion, and equal opportunity in the armed services: Background and issues for Congress*. Washington, DC: Congressional Research Service. Retrieved from https://fas .org/sgp/crs/natsec/R44321.pdf.

Kamareck, K. N., Mendez, B. H., & Library of Congress Washington DC (2021). *Military suicide prevention and response*. Washington, DC: Congressional Research Service.

Karney, B. R., & Crown, J. S. (2007). *Families under stress: An assessment of data, theory, and research on marriage and divorce in the military* (Vol. 599). Santa Monica, CA: RAND Corporation.

Keeling, M., Borah, E. V., Kintzle, S., Kleykamp, M., & Robertson, H. C. (2020). Military spouses transition too! A call to action to address spouses' military to civilian transition. *Journal of Family Social Work*, 23(1), 3–19.

Kim, J. B., Kirchhoff, M., & Whitsett, S. (2011). Expressive arts group therapy with middle-school aged children from military families. *The Arts in Psychotherapy*, 38(5), 356–362. https://doi.org/10.1016/j.aip.2011.08.003.

Koehlmoos, T. P., Korona-Bailey, J., Janvrin, M. L., & Madsen, C. (2022). Racial disparities in the military health system: A framework synthesis. *Military Medicine*, 187(9–10), e1114–e1121.

Kuz, M. (2019). For U.S. veterans, what does it mean to heal a moral injury? www.csmonitor.com/USA/Military/2019/1107/For-US-veterans-what-does-it-mean-to-heal-a-moral-injury.

LaCroix, J. M., Baer, M. M., Harrington-LaMorie, J., & Ghahramanlou-Holloway, M. (2018). Missed opportunities for military suicide prevention: Perspectives of suicide loss survivors. *Military Behavioral Health*, 6(3), 252–257. https://doi.org/10.1080/21635781.2017.1419893.

Lerner, R. M., Lerner, J. V., Geldhof, G. J., Gestsdóttir, S., King, P. E., Sim, A. T., & Dowling, E. (2018). Studying positive youth development in different nations: theoretical and methodological issues. In: J. E. Lansford & P. Banati (Eds.), *Handbook of adolescent development research and its impact on global policy*, Chapter 4, pp. 68–83. United Kingdom: Oxford University Press.

Lim, N. & Schulker, D. (2010). *Measuring underemployment among military spouses*. Santa Monica, Calif.: RAND Corporation.

Lim, N., Golinelli, D., & Cho, M. (2007). *"Working Around the Military" Revisited: Spouse Employment in the 2000 Census Data* (Vol. 566). Rand Corporation.

Linehan, M. M., & Wilks, C. R. (2015). The course and evolution of dialectical behavior therapy. *American Journal of Psychotherapy*, 69(2), 97–110.

Linsner, R. K., Maury, R. V., (2021, April). *Research brief: The impacts and opportunities of military life for military children*. Syracuse, NY: Institute for Veterans and Military Families, Syracuse University.

Litz, B. T., Lebowitz, L., Gray, M. J., Nash, W. P. (2016). *Adaptive disclosure: A new treatment for military trauma, loss, and moral injury*. United Kingdom: Guilford Publications.

Litz, B. T., Stein, N., Delaney, E., Lebowitz, L., Nash, W. P., Silva, C., & Maguen, S. (2009). Moral injury and moral repair in war veterans: A preliminary model and intervention strategy. *Clinical Psychology Review*, 29(8), 695–706.

Loughran, D. S. (2014). Why is veteran unemployment so high? Retrieved from www.rand.org/pubs/research_reports/RR284.html.

Lundgren, T., Luoma, J. B., Dahl, J., Strosahl, K., & Melin, L. (2012). The bull's-eye values survey: A psychometric evaluation. *Cognitive and Behavioral Practice*, 19(4), 518–526.

Maguen, S., Nichter, B., Norman, S. B., & Pietrzak, R. H. (2023). Moral injury and substance use disorders among US combat veterans: Results from the 2019–2020 National Health and Resilience in Veterans Study. *Psychological Medicine*, 53(4), 1364–1370.

Mancini, J. A., Martin, J. A., & Bowen, G. L. (2003). Community capacity. In T. Gullotta & M. Bloom (Eds.), *Encyclopedia of primary prevention and health promotion* (pp. 319–331). New York: Plenum Press.

Mansfield, A. J., Kaufman, J. S., Marshall, S. W., Gaynes, B. N., Morrissey, J. P., & Engel, C. C. (2010). Deployment and the use of mental health services among US Army wives. *New England Journal of Medicine*, 362(2), 101–109.

Marnocha, S. (2012). Military wives' transition and coping: Deployment and the return home. *International Scholarly Research Notices*.

Marshall, A. D., Panuzio, J., & Taft, C. T. (2005). Intimate partner violence among military veterans and active duty servicemen. *Clinical Psychology Review*, 25(7), 862–876.

Martin, R., & Young, J. (2010). Schema therapy. In: K. S. Dobson (Ed.), *Handbook of cognitive-behavioral therapies* (3rd edition), Chapter 10, pp. 317–346. New York: Guilford Press.

Maury, R., & Stone, B. (2014, February). *Military spouse employment report*. Syracuse, N.Y.: Institute for Veterans and Military Families. Accessed September 8, 2015: http://vets.syr.edu/wp-content/uploads/2014/02/MilitarySpouseEmploymentReport_2013.pdf.

McCubbin, H. I., & Patterson, J. M. (2014). The family stress process: The double ABCX model of adjustment and adaptation. In H. I. McCubbin & M. B. Sussman (Eds.), *Social stress and the family: Advances and developments in family stress therapy and research* (1st ed.). New York: Routledge. https://doi.org/10.4324/9781315804439.

McCubbin, H. I. & Patterson, J. M. (1983). The family stress process: The double ABCX model of adjustment and adaptation. *Marriage & Family Review* 6, 7–37.

Meadows, S. O., Engel, C. C., Collins, R. L., Beckman, R., Cefalu, M., Hawes-Dawson, J., Doyle, M., Kress, A. M., Sontag-Padilla, L., Ramchand, R., Williams, K. (2018). *2015 Department of Defense health related behaviors survey (HRBS)*. Santa Monica, CA: RAND Corporation.

Meadows, S. O., Griffin, B. A., Karney, B. R., & Pollak, J. (2016). Employment gaps between military spouses and matched civilians. *Armed Forces & Society*, 42(3), 542–561.

Millegan, J., Engel, C., Liu, X., & Dinneen, M. (2013). Parental Iraq/Afghanistan deployment and child psychiatric hospitalization in the U.S. military. *General Hospital Psychiatry*, 35(5), 556–560.

Miller, K. M., Kabat, M., Henius, J., & Van Houtven, C. H. (2015). Engaging, supporting, and sustaining the invisible partners in care: Young caregivers of veterans from the post-9/11 era. *North Carolina Medical Journal*, 76(5), 320–322.

Monson, C. M., Taft, C. T., & Freedman, S. J. (2009). Military-related PTSD and intimate relationships: From description to theory-driven research and intervention development. *Clinical Psychology Review*, 29(8), 707–714.

National Academies of Sciences, Engineering, and Medicine (2019). *Strengthening the military family readiness system for a changing American society*. Washington, DC: The National Academies Press. Retrieved from www.nap.edu/ catalog/25380/strengthening-the-military-family-readiness-system-for-a-changing-american-society.

Negrusa, B., & Negrusa, S. (2014). Home front: Post-deployment mental health and divorces. *Demography*, 51(3), 895–916.

Office of the Under Secretary of Defense for Personnel and Readiness (2018). Population representation in the military services: Fiscal year 2016 summary report. Retrieved from www.cna.org/pop-rep /2016/summary/summary.pdf.

Paul, K. I., & Moser, K. (2009). Unemployment impairs mental health: Meta-analyses. *Journal of Vocational Behavior*, 74(3), 264–282.

Perlick, D. A., Straits-Tröster, K., Dyck, D. G., Norell, D. M., Strauss, J. L., Henderson, C., Close, J., Berger, N., Bonuck, E. R., Taber, K. H., Kalvin, C., Dolber, T., & Cristian, A. (2011). Multifamily group treatment for veterans with traumatic brain injury. *Professional Psychology: Research and Practice*, 42(1), 70–78. https://doi.org/10.1037/a0022319.

Peterson, A., Bozzay, M., Bender, A., Monahan, M., & Chen, J. (2022). Those left behind: A scoping review of the effects of suicide exposure on veterans, service members, and military families. *Death Studies*, 46(5), 1176–1185. https://doi.org/10.1080/07481187.2020.1802628.

Pflieger, J. C., Richardson, S. M., Stander, V. A., & Allen, E. S. (2022). Risk and protective factors predictive of marital instability in U.S. military couples. *Journal of Family Psychology*, 36(5), 791–802. https://doi.org/10.1037/fam0000949.

Pietrzak, R. H., & Cook, J. M. (2013). Psychological resilience in older US veterans: Results from the national health and resilience in veterans study. *Depression and Anxiety*, 30(5), 432–443. www.pewresearch.org/fact-tank/2019/09/10/the-changing-profile-of-the-u-s-military/.

Putnam, R. D. (2015). Bowling alone: America's declining social capital. In R. T. LeGates, & F. Stout (Eds.), *The city reader* (pp. 188–196). London: Routledge.

Ragsdale, J. M., Kochert, J. F., & Beehr, T. A. (2021). News from the front: A monthly study on stress and social support during a military deployment to a war zone. *Journal of Occupational Health Psychology*, 26(4), 326–338. https://doi.org/10.1037/ocp0000278.

Ramchand, R., Tanielian, T., Fisher, M. P., Vaughan, C. A., Trail, T. E., Epley, C., … & Ghosh-Dastidar, B. (2014). *Hidden heroes: America's military caregivers*. Santa Monica, CA: RAND Corporation.

Reger M. A., Brenner L. A., du Pont A. (2022). Traumatic brain injury and veteran mortality after the war in Afghanistan. *JAMA* 5(2), e2148158. doi:10.1001/jamanetworkopen.2021.48158.

Rennie, R., & Landreth, G. (2000). Effects of filial therapy on parent and child behaviors. *International Journal of Play Therapy*, 9(2), 19–37.

Resick, P. A., Monson, C. M., & Chard, K. M. (2017). *Cognitive processing therapy for PTSD: A comprehensive manual*. New York: The Guilford Press.

Resick, P. A., Monson, C. M., & Chard, K. M. (2006). Cognitive processing therapy: Veteran/military version. *Clinical Psychology*, 74, 898–907.

Riegel, D. J. (2013). Closing the 90/10 loophole in the Highland Education Act: How to stop exploitation of veterans, protect American taxpayers, and restore market incentives to the for-profit college industry. *The George Washington Law Review*, 81, 259.

Robinette, J. W., Bostean, G., Glynn, L. M., Douglas, J. A., Jenkins, B. N., Gruenewald, T. L., & Frederick, D. A. (2021). Perceived neighborhood cohesion buffers COVID-19 impacts on mental health in a United States sample. *Social Science & Medicine*, 285, 114269.

Runge, C. E., Waller, M., MacKenzie, A., & McGuire, A. C. (2014). Spouses of military members' experiences and insights: Qualitative analysis of responses to an open-ended question in a survey of health and wellbeing. *PloS one*, 9(12), e114755.

Ruiz, M., Scholes, S., & Bobak, M. (2018). Perceived neighbourhood social cohesion and depressive symptom trajectories in older adults: A 12-year prospective cohort study. *Social Psychiatry and Psychiatric Epidemiology* 53, 1081–1090. https://doi.org/10.1007/s00127-018-1548-4.

Ryan, C. & Siebens, J. (2012, February). *Educational attainment in the United States: 2009*. Washington, D.C.: United States Census Bureau, P20–566. www.census.gov.edgekey-staging.net/content/dam/Census/library/publications/2012/demo/p20-566.pdf.

Scott, D. L., Whitworth, J. D., & Herzog, J. R. (2017). *Social work practice with military populations*. Pearson.

Seligman, M. E. P. (2002). *Authentic happiness: Using the new positive psychology to realize your potential for lasting fulfillment*. New York: Free Press.

Shay, J. (2010). *Achilles in Vietnam: Combat trauma and the undoing of character*. New York: Simon and Schuster.

Shay, J. (2002). *Odysseus in America: Combat trauma and the trials of homecoming*. New York: Simon and Schuster.

Sher, L. (2021). The prevention of suicide among military veterans during the COVID-19 pandemic. *European Archives of Psychiatry and Clinical Neuroscience*, 271(2), 405–406. https://doi.org/10.1007/s00406-020-01217-9.

Sherman, M. D., & Fischer, E. P. (2012). Provider, veteran, and family perspectives on family education in Veterans Affairs community-based outpatient facilities. *Psychological Services*, 9(1), 89–100. https://doi.org/10.1037/a0027103.

Siegel, B. S., Davis, B. E., & Committee on Psychosocial Aspects of Child and Family Health and Section on Uniformed Services. (2013). Health and mental health needs of children in US military families. *Pediatrics*, 131(6), e2002–e2015.

Silvestrini, M., & Chen, J. A. (2023). "It's a sign of weakness": Masculinity and help-seeking behaviors among male veterans accessing posttraumatic stress disorder care. *Psychological Trauma: Theory, Research, Practice, and Policy*, 15(4), 665–671. https://doi.org/10.1037/tra0001382.

Smith, W. A., Allen, W. R., & Danley, L. L. (2007). "Assume the position … you fit the description": Psychosocial experiences and racial battle fatigue among African American male college students. *American Behavioral Scientist*, 51(4), 551–578.

Smith Slep, A. M., Foran, H. M., & Heyman, R. E. (2014). An ecological model of intimate partner violence perpetration at different levels of severity. *Journal of Family Psychology*, 28(4), 470.

Snyder, T. D., & Dillow, S. A. (2015). *Digest of education statistics 2013 (NCES 2015–011)*. Washington, DC: National Center for Education Statistics, Institute of Education Sciences, U.S. Department of Education.

Sripada, R. K., Hannemann, C. M., Schnurr, P. P., Marx, B. P., Pollack, S. J., & McCarthy, J. F. (2018). Mental health service utilization before and after receipt of a service-connected disability award for PTSD: Findings from a national sample. *Health Services Research*, 53(6), 4565–4583.

Steger, M.F., & Park, C.L. (2012). The creation of meaning following trauma: Meaning making and trajectories of distress and recovery. In R. A. McMackin, E. Newman, J. M. Fogler, & T. M. Keane (Eds.), *Trauma therapy in context: The science and craft of evidence-based practice* (pp. 171–192). Washington, DC: American Psychological Association.

Stevens, A. H., & Schaller, J. (2011). Short-run effects of parental job loss on children's academic achievement. *Economics of Education Review*, 30(2), 289–299.

Stover, C. S., Easton, C. J., & McMahon, T. J. (2013). Parenting of men with co-occurring intimate partner violence and substance abuse. *Journal of Interpersonal Violence*, 28(11), 2290–2314.

Street, A. E., Gilman, S. E., Rosellini, A. J., Stein, M. B., Bromet, E. J., Cox, K. L., Colpe, L. J., Fullerton, C. S., Gruber, M. J., Heeringa, S. G., Lewandowski-Romps, L., Little, R. J., Naifeh, J. A., Nock, M. K., Sampson, N. A., Schoenbaum, M., Ursano, R. J., Zaslavsky, A. M., Kessler, R. C., & Army STARRS collaborators (2015). Understanding the elevated suicide risk of female soldiers during deployments. *Psychological Medicine*, 45(4), 717–726. https://doi.org/10.1017/S003329171400258X.

Sullivan, K. S., Hawkins, S. A., Gilreath, T. D., & Castro, C. A. (2021). Mental health outcomes associated with profiles of risk and resilience among US Army spouses. *Journal of Family Psychology*, 35(1), 33.

Taft, C. T., Creech, S. K., Gallagher, M. W., Macdonald, A., Murphy, C. M., & Monson, C. M. (2016). Strength at home couples program to prevent military partner violence: A randomized controlled trial. *Journal of Consulting and Clinical Psychology*, 84(11), 935.

Tanielian, T., Kathryn E. Bouskill, K. E., Rajeev Ramchand, R., Esther M. Friedman, E. M., Trail, T. E., & Angela Clague, A. (2017). *Improving support for America's hidden heroes: A military caregiver research blueprint*. Santa Monica, CA: RAND Corporation.

Temple, J., Miller, M. M., Banford Witting, A. & Kim, A. B. (2017). "We walk on eggshells": A phenomenological inquiry of wives' experiences of living with active-duty Marine husbands with PTSD. *Journal of Family Social Work*, 20(2), 162–181.

Tran, T. V., Canfield, J., & Chan, K. T. (2017). Differential association between unemployment status and mental health among veterans and civilians. *Social Work in Mental Health*, 15(4), 419–434.

Tran, L. D., Grant, D., & Aydin, M. (2016). *The mental health status of California veterans*. Los Angeles, CA: UCLA Center for Health Policy Research.

Treuer, D. (2019). *The heartbeat of Wounded Knee: Native America from 1890 to the present*. Riverhead Books.

Ursano R. J., Kessler R. C., Stein M. B., et al. (2016). Risk factors, methods, and timing of suicide attempts among US army soldiers. *JAMA Psychiatry*, 73(7):741–749. doi:10.1001/jamapsychiatry.2016.0600.

U.S. Citizenship and Immigration Services (USCIS) (2018, January 8). Naturalization through military service. Retrieved from www.uscis.gov /military/naturalization-through-military-service.

U.S. Citizenship and Immigration Services (2017, May 19). Naturalization Fact Sheet. Retrieved from www.uscis.gov /news/fact-sheets/naturalization-fact-sheet.

U.S. Department of Defense (2018). Personal communication of 2017 service member and spouse survey statistics to supplement statistics reported in 2017 demographics: Profile of the military community. Washington, DC.

U.S. Department of Defense (2015). Military accessions vital to national interest (MAVNI) recruitment pilot program. Washington, DC. Retrieved from https://dod.defense.gov /news/mavni-fact-sheet.pdf.

U.S. Department of Veterans Affairs (2021). www.mentalhealth.va.gov/docs/data-sheets/2021/2021-National-Veteran-Suicide-Prevention-Annual-Report-FINAL-9-8-21.pdf.

U.S. Department of Veteran Affairs (2018). Denied posttraumatic stress disorder claims related to military sexual trauma. Office of the Inspector General: Washington, DC. Retrieved from: www.va.gov/oig/pubs/VAOIG-17-05248-241.pdf.

U.S. Equal Employment Opportunity Commission (2020). Veterans and the Americans with Disabilities Act. Retrieved from: www.eeoc.gov/protections-against-employment-discrimination-service-members-and-veterans.

U.S. Government Accountability Office (2018). Military personnel: DoD should improve its oversight of the exceptional family member program. Washington, DC.

Van Ee, E., Murris, S., & Kool, D., (2018). We used to live on our own little islands: A qualitative evaluation of multifamily therapy with veterans. *Journal of Aggression, Maltreatment & Trauma*, 27(6), 689–702. https://doi.org/10.1080/10926771.2018.1473904.

Van Houtven, C. H., Friedemann-Sánchez, G., Clothier, B., Levison, D., Taylor, B. C., Jensen, A. C., et al. (2013). Is policy well-targeted to remedy financial strain among caregivers of severely injured U.S. service members? *Inquiry*, 49(4), 339–351.

Vaughan, C., Trail, T. E., Mahmud, A., Dellva, S., Tanielian, T., & Friedman, E. (2018). Informal caregivers' experiences and perceptions of a web-based peer support network: Mixed-methods study. *Journal of Medical Internet Research*, 20(8), https://doi.org/10.2196/jmir.9895.

Verdeli, H., Baily, C., Vousoura, E., Belser, A., Singla, D., & Manos, G. (2011). The case for treating depression in military spouses. *Journal of Family Psychology*, 25(4), 488.

Walsh, F. (2016). *Strengthening family resilience* (3rd ed.). New York, NY: Guilford.

Wang, M. C., Harcrow, A. M., Spears, A., & Nyutu, P. (2018). Affect, coping, and satisfaction with life among military spouses. *Military Behavioral Health*, 6(4), 346–354.

Weiss, E. L. & Castro C. A. (2019). *American military life in the 21st century: Social, cultural, and economic issues and trends*. Santa Barbara, CA. ABC-CLIO, LLC.

Weiss, E. L., Hino, D., Canfield, J., & Albright, D. L. (2016). Military families: Strengths and concerns: Reintegration and beyond. In J. Beder (Ed.), *Caring for the military: A guide for helping professionals* (pp. 72–92). New York: Routledge.

Weiss, E. L., Coll, J. E., Gerbauer, J., Smiley, K., & Carillo, E. (2010). The military genogram: A solution-focused approach for resiliency building in service members and their families. *The Family Journal*, 18(4), 395–406.

Wertsch, M. E. (2006). *Military brats: Legacies of childhood inside the fortress*. St. Louis, MO: Brightwell Publishing.

Whitesell, M., Bachand, A., Peel, J., & Brown, M. (2013). Familial, social, and individual factors contributing to risk for adolescent substance use. *Journal of Addiction*, 2013: 579310: 1–9. https://doi.org/10.1155/2013/579310.

Wilson, G., Hill, M., & Kiernan, M. D. (2018). Loneliness and social isolation of military veterans: Systematic narrative review. *Occupational Medicine*, 68(9), 600–609. https://doi.org/10.1093/occmed/kqy160.

Wolpert, D. S., Martin, J. A., Dougherty, L. M., Rudin, B. J., and Kerner-Hoeg, S. (2000). The special case of the young enlisted family. In J. A. Martin, L. N. Rosen, & L. R. Sparacino (Eds.),

The Military Family: A Practice Guide for Human Service Providers (pp. 43–53). Westport, Conn.: Praeger.

Wortmann, J. H., Nieuwsma, J. A., King, H. A., Fernandez, P., Jackson, G. L., Smigelsky, M. A., Cantrell, W., & Meador, K. G. (2022). Collaborative spiritual care for moral injury in the Veterans Affairs Healthcare System (VA): Results from a national survey of VA chaplains, *Journal of Health Care Chaplaincy*, 28 (sup1), S9–S24.

Yamada, A. M., Atuel, H. R., & Weiss, E. L. (2013). Military culture and multicultural diversity among military service members: Implications for mental health providers. In F. A. Paniagua & A. M. Yamada (Eds.), *Handbook of multicultural mental health* (2nd edition), (pp. 389–410). Academic Press.

Yambo, T. W., Johnson, M. E., Delaney, K. R., Hamilton, R., Miller, A. M., & York, J. A. (2016). Experiences of military spouses of veterans with combat-related posttraumatic stress disorder. *Journal of Nursing Scholarship*, 48(6), 543–551.

Young, J. E. (1990). *Cognitive therapy for personality disorders*. Sarasota, FL: Professional Resources Press.

Young, J. E., Arntz, A., Atkinson, T., Lobbestael, J., Weishaar, M. E., van Vreeswijk, M. F., et al. (2007). *The Schema Mode Inventory*. New York: Schema Therapy Institute.

Young, J. E., Klosko, J., & Weishaar, M. E. (2003). *Schema therapy: A practitioner's guide*. New York: Guilford Press.

Ziol-Guest, K., & Kalil, A. (2014). Frequent moves in childhood can affect later earnings, work, and education: The impact of childhood moves between ages 6 and 10 reverberates long into adulthood. *How Housing Matters*, pp. 1–4. Chicago, IL: John D. and Catherine T. MacArthur Foundation.

Index

Note: Locators in *italic* indicate figures and in ***bold italic*** boxes.

ABCX Theory / Double ABCX Theory family adaptation to stress 63–66, *63*, 69, 111, 149
active-duty mobility culture / military lifestyle 10–15; active-duty service members, numbers and locations 11; childhood/adolescence impact (*see* adolescence; child development and military lifestyle); economic impact, concerns 13; PCS frequency 12–13; relocation frequency 12; relocation orders (PCS, TDY) 11, 12–13, 18–19, 42, 73, 100, 129; social relationships, conflict resolution needs/ability 18; *see also* military culture
adaptive / maladaptive coping (strategies, skills) 21, 38, 42, 53, 54, 59, 62, 140
adaptive disclosure 127
ADHD (attention-deficit hyperactivity disorder) 35, ***46***
adolescence 12; alcohol and substance abuse 61–62; core values 44; community support capacity 65; Double ABCX Theory/studies 64–65; friendships, forming/retaining 13; maladaptive coping and depression 62–63; mental health 62–63, 92, 139–140; media accuracy trust 64–65; Positive Youth Development (PYD) model 43–45, *44*; resiliency 41–42; risk factors 61–63; social conflict resolution needs/ability 13, 18; transition experience 138–140; *see also* child development and military lifestyle
affect management 67, 81–83, 103
alcohol / alcohol abuse 20, 52, 61–63, 86, 119, 128, 134; *see also* substance use
ambiguous boundaries 67–71
ambiguous loss 68–71; attachment bonds, attachment security 67–68; children and 71; concept 68, 69; dealing with, treatment 69–70; denial 68; and family boundary ambiguity 69; family narrative creation 70; impact 68–69; psychological family 68; trauma exposure, traumatic stress 67, 69
Army Spouse Employment Partnership 76
attachment, styles/pattern 42, 66–67, 68, 70, *102*; and ambiguous loss management 67–68; assessment 99; attachment security/anxiety 42, 67–68, 88, 96–97, 103, 118–119, 123; avoidance 66, 83, *102*, 116, 118, 122; mistrust, interpersonal violence 88; strengthening (trauma-informed care model) *101–102*, 101–103, 124; trauma impact 82, 88, *101–102*, 101–103
attachment bonds, children: adult life impact 82, 88; ambiguous loss 71; attachment-focused family therapy 98; attunement behaviors 98, 99, ***104***; communication habit pattern 96–97; conflict resolution skills and attachment bond maintaining 41; developmental needs 37; filial play therapy 98–99; outside family 41; parental mental health challenges, impact 92; parent–child 66–67, 96–100, 118
attachment system, family as 66–67
attachment theory 66–67, 66–76
attachment-focused family therapy 98
attunement behaviors 98, 99, ***104***
autism 35

Battleground Mindset 47
belonging, sense of 19, 21–22, 27, 42, 68, 77, 129
Boss, P. 68–69
boundary ambiguity 68–71
Bowlby, J. 65–66

Caregivers and Veterans Omnibus Health Services Act (2010) 78
case examples: ambiguous loss coping as parenting challenges ***71–72***; Drako Family: pre-deployment (stable home life) 154–156 / deployment phase (loss, upheaval) 156–157 / post-deployment (family accommodation to change) 157–159; family adjustment and stress model adaptation ***89–91***; military medical retirement ***134–135***; military spouses, adaptability ***29–30***; notification order response ***46***; Solution-Focused Brief Therapy (SFBT) ***104–105***; veterans and civilian employment challenges ***150–151***
child development and military lifestyle 40–43; active-duty children, demographics 7, 40; active-duty vs National Guard and Reserve families 18, 40–41; adverse life events,

chronic stress/trauma 32; ambiguous loss, boundary ambiguity 68–71; attachment bonds (*see* attachment bonds, children); conflict resolution skills 41; deployment separation and transition experience/response 8, 110, 137–139; developmental attachment challenges 37; education disruption 12, 13–14, 138; friendships, forming/retaining 13; parental traumatic stress, impact 103; parent-focused families, impact 34, 36–38, 39, 40, 139–140; parenting styles 37–38; resilience characteristics *97–98*; role model 8, 41, 65, *65*; schemas, coping styles 38–40; special needs 35–36
climate, organizational 20–21, 26, 27
clinical education 142–144
closed ranks families *65*
Cognitive Processing Therapy (CPT) 103–104
collaborative problem solving 84, 85, 97, ***104–105***, 116
collectivist perspective 22, 28, 50, 110, 141, 150
Combat Operational Stress Continuum Model (COSC) 47
communication: break down, impact 67, 83–84; case example: ambiguous loss coping as parenting challenges 71–72; as comforting factor, deployment danger perception 79; as resiliency skills 50, 65–66, 82–83, 84; Solution-Focused Brief Therapy (SFBT) 41, 47, 100–101, 103–104, ***104–105***; styles 81–82, 84
community: climate, organizational 26–27, 28; community support capacity, resiliency/stress management 31–32, 55–56, 65, 86; interpersonal violence (IPV), community-level support 86; military, unifying nature (*see* military culture); PTSD/traumatic stress, community-based treatment approach 118–119, 129–130; relocation support 139; separation and loss 80–81
Community Capacity-Building Practice Model *65*
concussion 94–95, *95*, 96, 145
coping (adaptive, maladaptive) 21, 38, 42, 53, 54, 59, 62, 140
coping styles 38–40
core values 18, 19, 31, 50–51, 52, 53–54
crisis; *see* family crisis
cultural competency 15, 24–25, *25*, 142
cultural humility 15, 24–26, *25*, 153–154
culture, organizational 26–27, 28
customs, standard behavior 19, 26, 27, 52

demographic characteristics: active-duty children 7; active-duty and reserve service member 8–9; active-duty service members, numbers and locations 11; age 10–11; education, pre-enlistment 10; gender, sexuality 9; marital and parental status 8; non-citizens 11; racial and ethnic diversity 8–9; spouses 9–10
depression 34, 47, 62, 80, 95; case examples: ambiguous loss coping as parenting challenges *71–72*; military medical retirements ***134–135***; *see also* mental health
Double ABCX Theory 63–66, *63*, 69, 111, 149

Ebaugh, H. R. F. 60
employment, veteran 78, 112, 148–149; case example: John 150–151
employment opportunity lack, spouses 77–78, 137
Erikson, E. H. 43
ethos, military 17, 52, 55, 116, 150
Exceptional Family Member Program (EFMP) 35

Family Advocacy Program (FAP) 87
family crisis: adaptation ability, family characteristics ***65***; collaborative problem solving 84, 85, 97, ***104–105***, 116; in deployment 83–85; determinants, identifying 54–55, 64, 83; values/beliefs and crisis resiliency 18, 31, 49–50
Family Readiness Groups 23, 33
Family Readiness Support 7
family resilience: adversity as challenge mindset 110; attachment security / attachment system, and stress coping 66–67, 97; beliefs, core values 49–50; collectivist mentality 110; communication, affect management 50, 79–82, 84, 97; characteristics, adapting to wartime service *65*; deployment separation/loss 33, 62, 70, 79, 117; military culture internalization 15–16, 42 (*see also* military culture); measuring 51–55; organizational patterns 50; parent–child attachments 66–67, 96–100, 118; resilience training (Battleground Mindset, Military One Source) 11, 24, 47, 77, 86; Self-Assessment for Military Family Resiliency 152; *see also* child development and military lifestyle
filial play therapy 98–99
fortress, active-duty military as 21, *22*

General Allotment Act (1887) 111
G.I. Bill (1944) 112–113, 145
group (identity, affiliation, cohesion) 11, 16–17, 19, 22, 25–26, 27, 28, 48, 110

Hall, L. K. 21, 37

Indian Removal Act (1830) 111
interpersonal violence (IPV) 86–89; community level support 86; defining 86; ecological model for IPV 86; Family Advocacy Program (FAP) 87; military hierarchical culture, influence 87; Military OneSource program 11, 24, 47, 77, 86; rates 86–87; reporting 87; risk factors 86; splitting as trauma response 88; "Strength at Home for Couples" program 88–89

Koehlmoos, T. P. 111

language, common 18–19, 25
Lerner, J. V. *44*
Lerner, R. M. *44*

maladaptive / adaptive coping (strategies, skills) 21, 38, 42, 53, 54, 59, 62, 140
maladaptive schemas 38, 39, 40
Martin, R. 40
McCubbin, H. I. 63, 111
measuring resilience, Walsh Family Resilience Questionnaire 51, 54–55
mental health: adolescence 62–63, 92, 139–140; case examples: ambiguous loss coping as parenting challenges *71–72*; military medical retirements ***134–135***; Cognitive Processing Therapy (CPT) 103–104; comorbidity 95, *96*; depression 34, 47, 62, 80, 95; military mobility impact (treatment interruptions/terminations) 129, 139 moral injury (*see* moral injury); PTSD (*see* Post-Traumatic Stress Disorder (PTSD)); sexual assault and trauma 93; Solution-Focused Brief Therapy (SFBT) 41, 47, 100–101, 103–104, ***104–105***; spouses 34, *35*; stigma 128, 130; suicide 131–134; traumatic brain injuries (TBI) 94–96, *95*; unemployment 149; veterans 142–143, 153
Military Child Education Coalition 21
military culture 15–23; active-duty vs National Guard and Reserve families 17; belonging, sense of 19, 21–22, 27, 42, 68, 77, 129; case example: group identity, belonging ***29–30***; vs civilian culture 22–23; core values 18, 19, 31, 50–51, 52, 53–54; cultural pattern, behavioral expectations 17; customs, standard behavior 19, 26, 27, 52; ethos 17, 52, 55, 116, 150; family as part 15–16; group identity/affiliation (inward, outward) 11, 16–17, 19, 22, 25–26, 27, 28, 48, 110; historical development 15–16; language, common 18–19, 25; military installations as shared living environment 17, 19; need fulfillment, military-over-family 20; perpetual war threat 15; social characteristics 21–22; social fortress, active-duty military as 21, *22*; virtues, codes of conduct 21–23; warrior society / warrior identity 21–22, *22*, 27, 113–114, 116, 141, 147, 150
military family life cycle 7
military family support, professionalization 7
Military Family Timeline 53–54
Military Family Triangle 33–34, *35*
Military Genogram 51–53
military medical retirement 113, ***134–135***, 141–142
Military OneSource 11, 24, 47, 77, 86
Military Spouse Preference program 77
military-to-civilian transition (MCT) 136
military transition theory (MTT) 137
mobility; *see* active-duty mobility culture

moral injury 125–128; adaptive disclosure as treatment approach 127; care, treatment 126–127; civilian therapists training 127, 153–154; concept, symptoms, sources 125–126; diagnosis 125–126, 127; family impact 127–128, 137; health outcome 127–128; and PTSD (differences, co-morbidity) 125, 133; redemption acts 127–128; in war context 125–126, 127

National Guard and Reserve (NG/R) 17–18, 23–24, 28, 40, 62, 77, 114, 133, 150

organizational climate 20–21, 26, 27
organizational culture 26–27, 28

parenting: absence 21, *22*, 23, 28, 64; adolescents, risk factors 61–62; affect regulation problems 103; case examples: ambiguous loss coping as parenting challenges *71–72*; coercive parenting 37; deployment-related role shifts 64, 92–93; parental mental health, impact 92, 103; parent–child attachment 66–67, 96–100, 110, 118; parenting styles 37–38; permissive parenting 38; respectful leadership parenting 38; school changes; adapting ***46***; single 74, 79, 92; *see also* ambiguous loss; ambiguous boundaries
parent-focused families 34, 36–38, 39, 40, 139–140
partial PTSD 119; *see also* Post-Traumatic Stress Disorder (PTSD)
Patterson, J. M. 63, 111
Permanent Change of Station (PCS) 11, 12–13, 18–19, 42, 100, 129
Persistent Post-Concussive Symptoms (PPCS) 95, *95*
Persistent Post-Concussive Syndrome (PPCS) 95, *95*
Positive Youth Development (PYD) model 43–45, *44*
Post-Traumatic Stress Disorder (PTSD): case example: John, veteran ***150–151***; case example: Staff Sgt. Samuels ***134–135***; Cognitive Processing Therapy (CPT) 103–104, 130; community-based treatment approach 129–130; concept, symptoms 125; co-occurring mental health concerns 94–96, *95*; demographics 123; family caregiving 130; full and partial 119; lifetime disability rating for PTSD 130, ***134–135***; and moral injury (differences, co-morbidity) 125, 133; and Persistent Post-Concussive Syndrome (PPCS) 95, *95*; prevention programs 130; spousal/family experience and accommodation 82, 103–104, 115, 123–124, 128–130; and traumatic brain injury (TBI) overlap 95–96, *95*; treatment 103–104, 120, 128–130

post-traumatic stress (PTS); *see* traumatic/post-traumatic stress
predominantly White institutions (PWI) 146
psychological family 68

racial and ethnic diversity, service personal/military families 8–9
racial and ethnic veterans, unemployment rates 148
racial/ethnic minority student veterans 146
racism 111–113; employment rate differences 148; higher education 112, 146; home ownership 113; income and retirement benefits 113; institutionalized, systemic 25–26, 32–33, 111, 113; leadership roles 25–26; microaggressions 111, 146; military ranks 111, 113; Native American 111, 112; predominantly White institutions (PWI), support lack in 146; *see also* cultural competency and cultural humility
Rehabilitation Act (ADA, 1973) 36, ***151***
resiliency 31–33, 47–48, 49–50, 111–113; beliefs and core values 49–50, 50–51; child and youth development 31–32, 41–42, 43–45, ***97–98***; clinical education, policy change 142–144; communication styles and capacity 50–51, 55–56, 65–66, 82–83, 84 (*see also* communication); concept 32; core beliefs and values 18, 19, 31, 42, 50–51, 52, 53–54; management, community capacity 31–32, 55–56; markers 31–33; measuring tools 51–55, 152–153; Military Family Timeline 42, 53–54; Military Family Triangle 33–34, *35*; Military Genogram 51–53; organizational pattern 50; psychosocial functioning attributes 41–42; risk factors 42; special needs 35–36; stress management capacity, assessing 47–56; task-oriented and emotion-focused coping 21, 47–49, 88; *see also* Post-Traumatic Stress Disorder (PTSD); traumatic/post-traumatic stress
role exit / Role Exit Theory 59–60
roles, combat: civilian warriors, NG/R 23–24; female service member 23; male-only conscription 23
roles in families/military couples: allocation 8; boundary ambiguity, ambiguous loss 68, 70; confusion *122*; deployment cycle (shifts, renegotiation, confusion) 8, 15, 33, 50, 60–61; Double ABCX Theory 63–64; role model 8, 41, 65, ***65***
Rostker v. Goldberg (1981) 23

schemas / schema therapy model 38–40
secondary traumatic stress (STS) 114, 119–123, *121–122*, 124, *124*
sexual assault 93–94, 131
Solution-Focused Brief Therapy (SFBT) 41, 47, 100–101, 103–104, ***104–105***
special needs 35–36
Spouse Education and Career Opportunities (SECO) *76–77*
spouses ***134–135***; civilian careers 73–78; demographic characteristics 9–10; intimate partner violence 86; labor force penalty, employment lack 77–78, 137; mental health 34, *35*; Military Family Triangle, military-over-family priority response 34–35, 42; resilience risk and protective factors 34, *35*; role exit, role changes 60, 61; transition experience, "Military Spouses Transition Too!" report 136–139; as veteran care givers 78, 130
"Strength at Home for Couples" program 88–89
stress adaptation 59–72; affect regulation skills 67, 81–83, 103; ambiguous loss handling (*see* ambiguous loss); attachment system 65–66; boundary ambiguity risks 68–71; Double ABCX Theory 63–66, *63*, 69, 111, 149; family characteristics 65–66, ***65***; role exit, Role Exit Theory 59–61
stress and resilience 31–33, 47–48, 49–50, 111–113; beliefs and core values 49–50, 50–51; child development 31–32, 41–42, ***97–98***; communication 50–51; core values 49–50; management, community capacity 31–32, 55–56; measuring resiliency, tools 51–55, 152–153; organizational pattern 50; stress management capacity assessment 47–56; task-oriented and emotion-focused coping 21, 47–49, 88; *see also* Post-Traumatic Stress Disorder (PTSD); traumatic/post-traumatic stress
subjugation schema 39, 40
substance use 20, 52, 61–62, 86, 92, 95, 128, 134
suicide 128, 131–134, 143

Temporary Duty Yonder (TDY) 11, 73
transgender 10
trauma and attachment 82, 88, *101–102*, 101–103
trauma-focused family therapy *101–102*, 101–103
traumatic brain injuries (TBI) 94–96, *95*
traumatic/post-traumatic stress 109–124; associated complications, families *124*; Cognitive Processing Therapy (CPT) 103–104; family impact and family therapy *101–102*, 101–103; inter-generational 41; military adolescents substance use 62–63; posttraumatic / PTSD (*see* Post-Traumatic Stress Disorder (PTSD)); racism and military service 111–113; resilience and stress 109–111; secondary 114, 119–123, *121–122*, 124, *124*; social support 111; symptoms 96; triggers, environmental and internal ***124***; unresolved childhood trauma 82–83; wartime separation, changes 109

Uniform Code of Military Justice 21, 86

Vet Centers 143
veterans: case examples: Army Staff Sargent Samuels, military medical retirements

134–135 / John, veterans and civilian employment challenges ***150–151***; civilian life challenges 146–148; Department of Veterans Affairs loans 113; employment and well-being 78, 112, 148–149; ethnic/minority veterans 112–113; families/spouses as care givers 78, 130; family narratives renewal 149–150; G.I. Bill 112–113, 145; health treatments, care provision 2, 78; interpersonal/intimate partner violence 86, 88; military medical retirement 113, ***134–135***, 141–142; moral injury 125, 126, 127; racial/ethnic minority student veterans 146; resiliency through clinical education and policy change 142–144; students in higher education 112, 145–146; suicides 131, 132, 134; trauma-related stress, medical treatment, social support (PTSD, TBI) 94, 101, 103, 111, 114–116, 118–119, *121–122*, 123, 132–133
Veterans Health Administration (VHA) 142–143, 147–148
virtues 21–23

Walsh Family Resilience Questionnaire 51, 54–55
warrior identity/mindset 21–22, 27, 113–114, 116, 141, 147
warrior society 21, *22*, 150
Wertsch, M. E. 21

Yellow Ribbon Programs 145
yonder (Temporary Duty Yonder) 11, 73
Young, J. 40
youth development; *see* adolescence

9781032571768